DICTIONARY OF MEDICAL EMERGENCIES

English - Italian
Italian - English

DIZIONARIO DI EMERGENZE MEDICHE

Inglese – Italiano
Italiano - Inglese

Edita Ciglenečki

Copyright © 2016 Edita Ciglenečki
All rights reserved.
ISBN-13: 978-1540868589
ISBN-10: 1540868583

## INTRODUCTION - INTRODUZIONE

The audience for this dictionary includes medical professionals working in multilingual environments; global health professionals in tourist areas; professionals in public health, humanitarian medicine, emergency disaster management, rescue teams and above all, frequent travellers disposed to any kind of danger or health risk and therefore in the need of medical assistance while in some foreign speaking country. In emergency situations even small misunderstandings can lead to the loss of valuable time and consequently lives, therefore this English-Italian and Italian-English dictionary is created in very practical time-saving and easy-to-understand way for both medical professionals and their patients. Instead of one classical A to Z alphabetical order, it consists of over 3000 medical terms divided to several topics where terms regarding each topic are organized alphabetically. The topics start from very basic subjects of numbers and orientation and proceed with terminology concerning accidents and disasters, parts of the human body, injuries, symptoms and diseases, pharmacy, medical facilities, medical procedures, diagnostics, pregnancy and obstetrics.

Questo dizionario inglese-italiano ed italiano-inglese, contiene più di 3000 termini medici, ed è stato concepito come un manuale compatto di facile comprensione di terminologia medica dall'orientamento nel tempo e spazio; gli accidenti, catastrofi e angoscia; parti del corpo umano; i sintomi, ferite e malattie; farmacia; istituzioni, procedure e cure di medicina ed esami medici, alla gravidanza e ostetricia.

# CONTENTS – CONTENUTO

| | | |
|---|---|---|
| i | INTRODUCTION - INTRODUZIONE | 3 |
| ii | CONTENTS - CONTENUTO | 4 |
| iii | DICTIONARY OF MEDICAL EMERGENCIES / DIZIONARIO DI EMERGENZE MEDICHE | 5 |
| 1 | NUMBERS / NUMERI | 7 |
| 2 | ORIENTATION IN TIME / ORIENTAMENTO NEL TEMPO | 7 |
| 3 | ORIENTATION IN SPACE / ORIENTAMENTO NELLO SPAZIO | 7 |
| 4 | ACCIDENTS, CATASTROPHES AND DISTRESS / GLI ACCIDENTI, CATASTROFI E ANGOSCIA | 7 |
| 5 | PARTS OF THE HUMAN BODY / PARTI DEL CORPO UMANO | 9 |
| 6 | SYMPTOMS, INJURIES AND DISEASES / I SINTOMI, FERITE E MALATTIE | 13 |
| 7 | PHARMACY / FARMACIA | 37 |
| 8 | MEDICAL FACILITIES, PROCEDURES AND CARE / ISTITUZIONI, PROCEDURE E CURE DI MEDICINA | 39 |
| 9 | MEDICAL EXAMS / ESAMI MEDICI | 43 |
| 10 | PREGNANCY AND OBSTETRICS / GRAVIDANZA ED OSTETRICIA | 46 |
| iv | DIZIONARIO DI EMERGENZE MEDICHE / DICTIONARY OF MEDICAL EMERGENCIES | 49 |
| 1 | NUMÉRI / NUMBERS | 51 |
| 2 | ORIENTAMENTO NEL TEMPO / ORIENTATION IN TIME | 51 |
| 3 | ORIENTAMENTO NELLO SPAZIO / ORIENTATION IN SPACE | 51 |
| 4 | GLI ACCIDENTI, CATASTROFI E ANGOSCIA / ACCIDENTS, CATASTROPHES AND DISTRESS | 51 |
| 5 | PARTI DEL CORPO UMANO / PARTS OF THE HUMAN BODY | 53 |
| 6 | I SINTOMI, FERITE E MALATTIE / SYMPTOMS, INJURIES AND DISEASES | 57 |
| 7 | FARMACIA / PHARMACY | 81 |
| 8 | ISTITUZIONI, PROCEDURE E CURE DI MEDICINA / MEDICAL FACILITIES, PROCEDURES AND CARE | 84 |
| 9 | ESAMI MEDICI / MEDICAL EXAMS | 87 |
| 10 | GRAVIDANZA ED OSTETRICIA / PREGNANCY AND OBSTETRICS | 90 |
| v | ABOUT THE AUTOR | 93 |

# DICTIONARY OF MEDICAL EMERGENCIES

English - Italian

# DIZIONARIO DI EMERGENZE MEDICHE

Inglese – Italiano

| NUMBERS | NUMERI |
|---|---|
| Zero | Zero |
| One | Uno |
| Two | Due |
| Three | Tre |
| Four | Quattro |
| Five | Cinque |
| Six | Sei |
| Seven | Sette |
| Eight | Otto |
| Nine | Nove |
| Ten | Dieci |
| Eleven | Undici |
| Twelve | Dodici |
| Thirteen | Tredici |
| Fourteen | Quattordici |
| Fifteen | Quindici |
| Sixteen | Sedici |
| Seventeen | Diciassette |
| Eighteen | Diciotto |
| Nineteen | Diciannove |
| Twenty | Venti |
| Twenty-one | Ventuno |
| Twenty-two | Ventidue |
| Thirty | Trenta |
| Forty | Quaranta |
| Fifty | Cinquanta |
| Sixty | Sessanta |
| Seventy | Settanta |
| Eighty | Ottanta |
| Ninety | Novanta |
| Hundred | Cento |
| One hundred and one | Centouno |
| One hundred and twenty-three | Centoventitre |
| Twohundred | Duecento |
| Three hundred | Trecento |
| Four hundred | Quattrocento |
| Five hundred | Cinquecento |
| Six hundred | Seicento |
| Seven hundred | Settecento |
| Eight hundred | Ottocento |
| Nine hundred | Novecento |
| Thousand | Mille |
| Two thousand | Duemila |
| Million | Un milione |
| Milliard (billion) | Un miliardo |

| ORIENTATION IN TIME | ORIENTAMENTO NEL TEMPO |
|---|---|
| Yesterday | Ieri |
| Today | Oggi |
| Tomorrow | Domani |
| Year | Anno |
| Month | Mese |
| Week | Settimana |
| Day | Giorno |
| Hour | Ora |
| Minute | Minuto |
| Second | Secondo |
| Morning | Mattina |
| Afternoon | Pomeriggio |
| Evening | Sera |
| Night | Notte |

| ORIENTATION IN SPACE | ORIENTAMENTO NELLO SPAZIO |
|---|---|
| Up (above) | Su |
| Down (below) | In basso |
| Left | Sinistra |
| Right | Destra |
| In front | Davanti |
| Behind | Dietro |
| Inside | Dentro |
| Outside | Fuori |

| ACCIDENTS, CATASTROPHES AND DISTRESS | GLI ACCIDENTI, CATASTROFI E ANGOSCIA |
|---|---|
| ABC weapons | Armi nucleari, biologiche e chimiche (NBC) |
| Air attack | Incursione area |
| Airplane crash | Incidente aereo |
| Alarm | Allarme |
| Alarm signal | Segnale di allarme |
| Atomic bomb (A-bomb) | Bomba atomica (bomba A) |
| Atomic weapons | Arma atomica |
| Attack | Attaco |
| Avalanche | Valanga |
| Bacteria | Batterio |
| Biological weapon | Arma biologica |
| Bomb | Bomba |
| Bullet | Pallottola |
| Call for help | Chiamata di aiuto |
| Car accident | Incidente stradale |
| Cave | Grotta |
| Chemical pollution | Inquinamento chimico |
| Chemical weapon | Arma chimica |
| Civil defense | Difesa civile |
| Cobalt bomb | Bomba al cobalto (bomba gamma, bomba G) |
| Cold weapon | Arma bianca |
| Collision | Collisione |
| Conventional weapon | Arma convenzionale |
| Dirty bomb | Bomba sporca |
| Domestic accident | Infortunio domestico |
| Drowned person | Annegato |
| Drowning | Annegamento |
| Earthquake | Terremoto |
| Electric shock | Folgorazione (elettrocuzione) |
| Enriched uranium | Uranio arricchito |
| Epidemic | Epidemia |

| | |
|---|---|
| Explosion | Esplosione |
| Explosive | Esplosivo |
| Fall | Cadutta (cascata) |
| Fight | Combattimento |
| Fire | Fuoco |
| Fire (conflagration) | Incendio (fuoco) |
| Firearm | Arma da fuoco |
| Flood | Inondazione |
| Heat stroke | Colpo di calore |
| Helicopter (chopper) | Elicottero |
| "Help!" | "Aiuto!" |
| Hidrogen bomb (H-bomb) | Bomba all'idrogeno (bomba H) |
| Homicide (murder) | Omicidio (uccisione) |
| Hostage | Ostaggio |
| Human trafficking | Traffico di esseri umani |
| Hurricane | Uragano |
| Ice | Ghiaccio |
| Iceberg | Ghiacciaio |
| Icebreaker | Rompighiaccio |
| Invasion | Invasione |
| Kidnapping | Rapimento |
| Lake | Lago |
| Land | Terra |
| Land mine | Mina terrestre |
| Laser weapon | Armi laser |
| Lava | Lava |
| Lifebelt (lifebuoy) | Boa di salvataggio |
| Lifeboat | Scialuppa |
| Lifejacket (life vest) | Giubbotto di salvataggio |
| Marine salvage | Salvataggio navale |
| Mine | Mina |
| Mine clearance (demining) | Eliminazione di mine (sminamento) |
| Mine field | Campo minato |
| Mountain | Montagna |
| Naval mine | Mina navale |
| Neurotoxin | Neurotossina |
| Neutron bomb | Bomba al neutrone (bomba N) |
| Nuclear accident | Accidente nucleare |
| Nuclear waste (radioactive waste) | Scoria nucleare (scoria radioattiva) |
| Nuclear weapon | Arma nucleare |
| Nuclear weapons testing | Test nucleare |
| Occupational accident | Infortunio sul lavoro |
| Pandemic | Pandemia |
| Parachute | Paracadute |
| Physical assault | Attacco fisico |
| Pirate | Pirata |
| Pirate attack | Attacco dei pirati |
| Plutonium | Plutonio |
| Poison gas | Gas tossico |
| Radiation | Radiazione |
| Rape (violation) | Violenza sessuale |
| Refugee | Rifugiato |
| Refugee camp | Campo per rifugiati |
| Rescuer | Salvatore |
| River | Fiume |
| Robbery | Rapina |
| Rock | Roccia |
| Rope | Cordone |
| Ruins | Macerie (rovine) |
| Salvage | Salvataggio |
| Sand storm | Tempesta di sabbia |
| Sea | Mare |
| Sea ice | Banchisa (ghiaccio marino; banchiglia) |
| Search | Ricerca |
| Search and rescue dog | Cane da ricerca e salvataggio |
| Search and rescue team | Squadra di ricerca e salvataggio |
| Shark attack | Attacco di squalo |
| Shelter | Rifugio |
| Ship | Nave |
| Ship wreck | Relitto |
| Shrapnel | Shrapnel |
| Sinking of a ship | Affondamento della nave |
| Slavery | Schiavitù (prigionia) |
| Snow | Neve |
| Snow storm | Bufera di neve (nevicata) |
| SOS call | SOS richiesta |
| Storm | Tempesta |
| Stranding of a ship | Incaglio di nave |
| Strategic nuclear weapon | Arma nucleare strategica |
| Stroke (hit, blow) | Colpo (botta) |
| Suicide | Suicidio |
| Tactical nuclear weapon | Arma nucleare tattica |
| Terrorist | Terrorista |
| Terrorist attack | Attentato terroristico |
| Terrorist cell | Cellula terroristica |
| Thunderclap | Percossa dal fulmine |
| Tidal wave | Onda di marea |
| Traffic accident | Incidente di traffico |
| Tsunami | Tsunami |
| Typhoon | Tifone |
| Uranium | Uranio |
| Victim | Vittima |
| Virus | Virus |
| Volcanic eruption | Eruzione vulcanica |
| War | Guerra |
| Water | Acqua |
| Waterspout | Tromba marina |
| Weapon | Arma |
| Weapon of mass destruction | Arma di distruzione di massa |

| PARTS OF THE HUMAN BODY | PARTI DEL CORPO UMANO |
|---|---|
| Abdominal aorta | Aorta addominale |
| Abdominal oblique muscle | Musculo obliquo dell'addome |
| Abdominal wall | Parete addominale |
| Acetabulum | Cotile (acetabolo) |
| Acetylcholine | Acetilcolina |
| Acoustic nerve (vestibulocochlear nerve) | Nervo vestibolococleare (nervo stato-acustico) |
| Adam's apple | Pomo d'Adamo |
| Adductor muscle | Muscolo adduttore |
| Adenohypophysis | Adenoipofisi |
| Adrenal gland | Surrene |
| Adrenalin (adrenaline) | Adrenalina |
| Agglutinin | Agglutinine |
| Agglutinogen | Agglutinogeno |
| Albumin | Albumina |
| Aldosterone | Aldosterone |
| Alveolus | Alveolo |
| Amino acid | Amminoacido |
| Ammonia | Ammoniaca |
| Ankle joint | Caviglia |
| Antidiuretic hormone (vasopressin) | Ormone antidiuretico (vasopressina) |
| Anus | Ano |
| Anvil (incus) | Incudine |
| Aorta | Aorta |
| Aortic valve | Valvola semilunare aortica |
| Aponeurosis | Aponeurosi |
| Arachnoid mater | Aracnoide |
| Arm | Braccio |
| Armpit (axilla, underarm) | Ascella |
| Arteriole | Arteriola |
| Artery | Arteria |
| Articular capsule (joint capsule) | Capsula articolare |
| Astrocyte | Astrocita |
| Atrioventricular node | Nodo atrioventricolare |
| Auditory canal (ear canal) | Meato acustico esterno |
| Back | Schiena (dorso) |
| Bartholin's gland | Ghiandola di Bartolini |
| Basophil granulocyte | Granulocita basofilo |
| Belly (abdomen) | Addome (ventre, pancia) |
| Biceps brachii muscle | Muscolo bicipite brachiale |
| Biceps femoris muscle | Bicipite femorale |
| Bile duct | Coledoco |
| Bilirubin | Bilirubina |
| Blood | Sangue |
| Blood group | Gruppo sanguigno |
| Blood group A | Gruppo sanguigno A |
| Blood group AB | Gruppo sanguigno AB |
| Blood group B | Gruppo sanguigno B |
| Blood group 0 | Gruppo sanguigno 0 |
| Blood vessel | Vaso sanguigno |
| Body fluid | Fluido corporale |
| Bone | Osso |
| Bone marrow | Midollo osseo |
| Brachialis muscle | Muscolo brachiale |
| Brain | Cervello |
| Brain marrow | Midollo cerebrale |
| Brain stem | Tronco encefalico |
| Brain ventricle | Ventricolo cerebrale |
| Breast | Mammella |
| Breastbone (sternum) | Sterno |
| Bronchiole | Bronchiolo |
| Bronchus | Bronco |
| Bulbourethral gland (Cowper's gland) | Ghiandola bulbouretrale (ghiandola di Cowper) |
| Bundle of His | Fascio di His |
| Calcaneus | Calcagno |
| Calcitonin | Calcitonina |
| Calf | Polpaccio |
| Canal of Schlemm | Canale di Schlemm |
| Canine tooth | Canino |
| Capillary | Capillare |
| Carbohydrate | Carboidrato (glucide) |
| Cardiac atrium | Atrio |
| Cardiac muscle (myocardium) | Miocardio |
| Cardiac ventricle | Ventricolo cardiaco |
| Carpus | Carpo |
| Cartilage | Cartilagine |
| Cartilage ring | Anello cartilagineo |
| Catecholamine | Catecolamina |
| Cell | Cellula |
| Cementum | Cemento |
| Cerebellum | Cervelletto |
| Cerebral cortex | Corteccia cerebrale |
| Cerebrospinal fluid | Liquido cefalora-chidiano (liquor, liquido cerebrospinale) |
| Cerebrum (telencephalon) | Telencefalo (cervello) |
| Cheek | Guancia |
| Chest | Torace |
| Chin | Mento |
| Cholesterol | Colesterolo |
| Choroid | Coroide |
| Ciliary muscle | Muscolo ciliare |
| Clitoris | Clitoride |
| Coccygeal vertebra | Vertebra coccigea |
| Cochlea | Coclea |

| | |
|---|---|
| Collagen | Collagene |
| Collarbone (clavicle) | Clavicola |
| Cornea | Cornea |
| Coronary artery | Arteria coronaria |
| Corpus luteum | Corpo luteo |
| Corticosteroid | Corticosteroide |
| Corticosterone | Corticosterone |
| Corticotropin (adrenocorticotropic hormone) | Corticotropina (ormone adrenocorticotropo) |
| Cortisol | Cortisolo |
| Cortisone | Cortisone |
| Cranial nerve | Nervo cranico |
| Crown ofa tooth | Corona del dente |
| Deltoid muscle | Muscolo deltoide |
| Dendrite | Dendrite |
| Dental pulp | Polpa dentaria |
| Dentin | Dentina |
| Deoxyribonucleic acid (DNA) | Acido desossiribonucleico (DNA) |
| Diaphragm | Muscolo diaframma |
| Diencephalon | Diencefalo |
| Duodenum | Duodeno |
| Dura mater | Dura madre (pachimeninge) |
| Ear | Orecchio |
| Eardrum (tympanic membrane) | Timpano (membrana timpanica) |
| Earwax (cerumen) | Cerume |
| Ejaculatory duct | Dotto eiaculatore |
| Elastin | Elastina |
| Elbow | Gomito |
| Elbow joint | Articolazione del gomito |
| Electrolyte | Elettrolita |
| Eosinophil | Eosinofilo |
| Epididymis | Epididimo |
| Erythrocyte (red blood cell) | Eritrocita (globulo rosso) |
| Estradiol | Estradiolo |
| Estrogen | Estrogeno |
| Ethmoid bone | Osso etmoide |
| Eye | Occhio |
| Eye orbit | Orbita oculare |
| Eyeball | Bulbo oculare |
| Eyebrow | Sopracciglio |
| Eyelash | Ciglia |
| Eyelid | Palpebra |
| Face | Viso |
| Fallopian tube (oviduct) | Tuba di Falloppio |
| Fat | Lipidi |
| Fat tissue | Tessuto adiposo |
| Fibrin | Fibrina |
| Fibrinogen | Fibrinogeno |
| Fibroblast | Fibroblasto |
| Fibula (calf bone) | Perone (fibula) |
| Finger | Dito della mano |
| Foot | Piede |
| Forearm | Avambraccio |
| Forefinger | Dito indice |
| Forehead | Fronte |
| Foreskin (prepuce) | Prepuzio |
| Frontal bone | Osso frontale |
| Gall (bile) | Bile |
| Gall bladder | Cistifellea |
| Gas | Gas |
| Gastric acid | Acido gastrico |
| Gastric juice | Succo gastrico |
| Gastric mucous membrane | Mucosa gastrica |
| Gland | Ghiandola |
| Glans | Glande |
| Globulin | Globulina |
| Glomerulus | Glomerulo |
| Glucagon | Glucagone |
| Glucocorticoid | Glucocorticoide |
| Glucose | Glucosio |
| Gluteal muscle | Muscolo gluteo |
| Glycogen | Glicogeno |
| Gonadotrophin | Gonadotropina |
| Granulocyte | Granulocita |
| Groin | Inguine |
| Growth hormone (somatotrophin) | Somatotropina |
| Gullet (oesophagus) | Esofago |
| Gums (gingiva) | Gengiva |
| Hair | Pelo |
| Hair | Capelli |
| Hammer (malleus) | Martello |
| Hand | Mano |
| Hard palate | Palato duro (volta palatina) |
| Head | Testa |
| Heart | Cuore |
| Heart valve (cardiac valve) | Valvola cardiaca |
| Heel | Tallone |
| Hemoglobin | Emoglobina |
| Hip bone | Osso dell'anca |
| Hip joint | Articolazione dell'anca |
| Hormone | Ormone |
| Hymen | Imene |
| Hyoid bone (lingual bone) | Osso ioide |
| Hypophysis (pituitary gland) | Ipòfisi (ghiandola pituitaria) |
| Hypothalamus | Ipotalamo |
| Ileum | Ileo |
| Ilium | Osso iliaco |
| Immunoglobulin | Immunoglobulina |
| Incisor | Incisivo |
| Inferior vena cava | Vena cava inferiore |
| Innominate bone (pelvis) | Bacino |
| Insulin | Insulina |
| Intercostal muscle | Muscolo intercostale |
| Interstitial fluid | Liquido extracellulare |
| Intervertebral disc | Disco intervertebrale |
| Intestinal juice | Succo intestinale |

| | |
|---|---|
| Intestinal villus | Villo intestinale |
| Intestine | Intestino |
| Iris | Iride |
| Ischium | Ischio |
| Jaw | Scheletro della bocca |
| Jejunum | Digiuno |
| Joint | Articolazione |
| Joint cartilage | Cartilagine articolare |
| Keratin | Cheratina |
| Kidney | Rene |
| Knee | Ginocchio |
| Kneecap (patella) | Rotula (patella) |
| Lachrymal bone | Osso lacrimale |
| Lachrymal gland | Ghiandola lacrimale |
| Large intestine (colon) | Intestino crasso (colon) |
| Larynx | Laringe |
| Leg | Arto inferiore |
| Lens | Cristallino |
| Leukocyte | Leucocita |
| Ligament | Legamento |
| Lip | Labbro |
| Little finger (pinky) | Mignolo |
| Liver | Fegato |
| Loin | Lombo |
| Lower jaw (mandible) | Mandibola |
| Lower leg | Gamba |
| Lumbar vertebra | Vertebra lombare |
| Lung | Polmone |
| Lungs | Polmoni |
| Luteinising hormone | Ormone luteinizzante |
| Lymph | Linfa |
| Lymph gland (lymph node) | Linfonodo |
| Lymph vessel | Vaso linfatico |
| Lymphocyte | Linfocita |
| Masseter muscle | Muscolo massetere |
| Medulla oblongata | Bulbo (midollo allungato, encefalo) |
| Melanin | Melanina |
| Melanotropin | Ormone melanotropo |
| Melatonin | Melatonina |
| Meninx | Meninge |
| Meniscus | Menisco |
| Metacarpal bone | Osso metacarpale |
| Metacarpus | Metacarpo |
| Metatarsal bone | Osso metatarsale |
| Metatarsus | Metatarso |
| Middle ear | Orecchio medio |
| Middle finger | Dito medio |
| Milk tooth | Dente da latte |
| Mineralcorticoid | Mineralcorticoide |
| Mitral valve (bicuspid valve) | Valvola mitrale (valvola bicuspide) |
| Molar | Molare |
| Monocyte | Monocita |
| Mouth | Bocca |
| Mouth cavity (oral cavity) | Cavità orale |
| Mucous membrane | Membrana mucosa |
| Mucus | Muco |
| Muscle | Muscolo |
| Muscular fascia | Fascia muscolare |
| Nail | Unghia |
| Nape (occiput) | Nuca |
| Nasal bone | Osso nasale |
| Nasolacrimal duct (tear duct) | Canale naso-lacrimale |
| Navel (belly button) | Ombelico |
| Neck | Collo |
| Nerve | Nervo |
| Nipple | Capezzolo |
| Noradrenaline | Noradrenalina |
| Nose | Naso |
| Nostril | Narice |
| Occipital bone | Osso occipitale |
| Optic nerve | Nervo ottico |
| Organ | Organo |
| Ovary | Ovaia |
| Ovum | Uovo |
| Oxytocin | Ossitocina |
| Palate | Palato |
| Palatine bone | Osso palatino |
| Palm | Palmo |
| Pancreas | Pancreas |
| Pancreatic juice | Succo pancreatico |
| Parasympathetic nervous system | Sistema nervoso parasimpatico |
| Parathyroid gland | Paratiroide |
| Parathyroid hormone | Paratormone (ormone paratiroideo) |
| Parietal bone | Osso parietale |
| Parietal pleura | Pleura parietale |
| Pectoralis major muscle | Muscolo grande pettorale |
| Pectoralis minor muscle | Muscolo piccolo pettorale |
| Penis | Pene |
| Pericardium | Pericardio |
| Perineum | Perineo |
| Peritoneum | Peritoneo |
| Phalanx bone | Falange |
| Pharynx (gullet, gorge) | Faringe |
| Phospholipid | Fosfolipide |
| Pia mater | Pia madre |
| Pineal body (pineal gland, epiphysis) | Ghiandola pineale (epifisi) |
| Pinna (auricle) | Padiglione auricolare |
| Plasma | Plasma |
| Pleura | Pleura (pleure) |
| Pore | Poro |
| Portal vein | Vena porta |
| Premolar | Premolare |
| Progesterone | Progesterone |
| Prostate | Prostata |
| Protein | Proteina |
| Pubis (pubic bone) | Pube (osso pubico) |
| Pulmonary artery | Arteria polmonare |
| Pupil | Pupilla |

| | |
|---|---|
| Quadriceps femoris muscle | Muscolo quadricipite femorale |
| Radius | Radio |
| Rectus abdominis muscle | Muscolo retto dell'addome |
| Retina | Rètina |
| Rh factor negative | Fattore Rh negativo |
| Rh factor positive | Fattore Rh positivo |
| Rhomboid muscle | Muscolo romboide |
| Rib | Costola (costa) |
| Rib cage | Gabbia toracica |
| Ribonucleic acid | Acido ribonucleico (ARN) |
| Ring finger | Anulare |
| Root of a tooth | Radice del dente |
| Sacral vertebra | Vertebra sacrale |
| Saliva (spit, slobber) | Saliva |
| Salivary gland | Ghiandola salivare |
| Scalp | Cuoio capelluto |
| Sclera | Sclera |
| Sebaceous gland | Ghiandola sebacea |
| Sebum | Sebo |
| Semen | Sperma |
| Semimembranosus muscle | Muscolo semimembranoso |
| Seminal vesicle | Vescicola seminale |
| Semitendinosus muscle | Muscolo semitendinoso |
| Sesamoid bone | Osso sesamoide |
| Sex gland (gonad) | Gonade |
| Shinbone (tibia) | Tibia |
| Shoulder | Spalla |
| Shoulder blade (scapula) | Scapola (omoplata) |
| Shoulder joint | Articolazione della spalla |
| Sigmoid colon | Sigma (colon sigmoideo) |
| Sinus | Seno |
| Skeleton | Scheletro |
| Skin | Pelle (cute) |
| Skull | Cranio |
| Skull base | Base del cranio |
| Small intestine | Intestino tenue (piccolo intestino) |
| Smooth muscle | Tessuto muscolare liscio |
| Soft palate | Palato molle |
| Sole | Pianta del piede |
| Sperm (spermatozoon) | Spermatozoo |
| Sphenoid bone | Osso sfenoide |
| Sphincter | Sfintere |
| Spinal cord | Midollo spinale |
| Spinal nerve | Nervo spinale |
| Spine (spinal column, backbone) | Columna vertebral |
| Spleen | Milza |
| Stirrup (stapes) | Staffa (columella) |
| Stomach | Stomaco |
| Stool (feces) | Feci |
| Striated muscle | Muscolo striato |
| Superior vena cava | Vena cava superiore |
| Sweat | Sudore |
| Sweat gland | Ghiandola sudoripara |
| Sympathetic nervous system | Sistema nervoso simpatico |
| Synapse | Sinapsi (bottone sinaptico) |
| Synovial bursa | Borsa sierosa |
| Synovial fluid (synovia) | Liquido sinoviale (sinovia) |
| Synovial membrane | Membrana sinoviale |
| Tailbone (coccyx) | Coccige |
| Tailor's muscle (sartorius muscle) | Muscolo sartorio |
| Tarsal bone | Osso tarsale |
| Tarsus | Tarso |
| Taste bud | Papilla gustativa |
| Tear | Lacrima |
| Temple | Tempia |
| Temporal bone | Osso temporale |
| Tendon (sinew) | Tendine |
| Testicle | Testicolo |
| Testosterone | Testosterone |
| Thalamus | Talamo |
| Thigh | Coscia |
| Thighbone (femur) | Femore |
| Thoracic aorta | Aorta toracica |
| Thoracic vertebra | Vertebra toracica |
| Throat | Gola |
| Thrombocyte | Trombocita (piastrina) |
| Thumb | Pollice |
| Thymus | Timo |
| Thyroid | Tiroide |
| Thyroid-stimulating hormone (TSH, thyrotropin) | Tirotropina (ormone tireostimolante) |
| Thyroxine | Tiroxina |
| Tissue | Tessuto |
| Toe | Dito del piede |
| Tongue | Lingua |
| Tonsil | Tonsille |
| Tooth | Dente |
| Tooth enamel | Smalto |
| Trapezius muscle | Muscolo trapezio |
| Triceps brachii muscle | Muscolo tricipite del braccio |
| Triceps surae muscle | Muscolo tricipite della sura |
| Tricuspid valve | Valvola tricuspide |
| Triglyceride | Trigliceride |
| Triiodothyronine | Triiodotironina |
| Trunk (torso) | Tronco |
| Tympanic cavity | Cassa del timpano |
| Ulna | Ulna (cubito) |
| Upper arm | Barccio |
| Upper arm bone (humerus) | Omero |
| Upper back | Schiena alto |
| Upper jaw (maxilla) | Osso mascellare |

| | |
|---|---|
| Urea | Urea |
| Ureter | Uretere |
| Urethra | Uretra |
| Urinary bladder | Vescica urinaria |
| Urine | Urina |
| Vagina | Vagina |
| Valve (valvula) | Valvola |
| Vein | Vena |
| Ventricle | Ventricolo |
| Venule | Venula |
| Vermiform appendix (cecal appaendix) | Appendice vermiforme |
| Vertebra | Vertebra |
| Vertex (crown of head) | Vertice della testa |
| Vestibule | Vestibolo |
| Visceral pleura | Pleura viscerale |
| Vocal chord | Corda vocale |
| Vomer | Vomere |
| Vulva | Vulva |
| Windpipe (trachea) | Trachea |
| Womb (uterus) | Utero |
| Wrist | Polso |
| Wrist bone (carpal bone) | Osso carpale |
| Zygoma (cheekbone, malar bone) | Osso zigomatico |

## SYMPTOMS, INJURIES AND DISEASES

## I SINTOMI, FERITE E MALATTIE

| | |
|---|---|
| Abdominal aortic aneurysm | Aneurisma dell'aorta addominale |
| Abdominal colic | Colica addominale |
| Abdominal pain | Dolore addominale |
| Abdominal wall tension | Tensione di parete addominale |
| Aberrant pancreas | Pancraes aberrante |
| Abnormal flexibility | Movimento anormale |
| Abnormal twisting of the intestines (volvulus) | Volvolo |
| Abnormally heavy menstrual period (menorrhagia) | Anormale perdita di sangue durante il ciclo mestruale (menorragia) |
| Abnormally large intake of food (hyperphagia) | Aumento incontrollato di assunzione di cibo (iperfagia) |
| Aboulia (disorder of diminished motivation) | Abulia |
| Abrasion | Abrasione (escoriazione) |
| Abscess | Ascesso |
| Absence in development of an organ (aplasia of an organ) | Mancato sviluppo di un organo (aplasia di un organo) |
| Absence of menstrual period (amenorrhea) | Assenza di mestruazioni (amenorrea) |
| Absence of pulse | Perdita di polso |
| Acariasis | Acariasi |
| Accelerated basal metabolism | Metabolismo basale accelerato |
| Accelerated pulse rate | Polso accelerato |
| Achilles tendon overuse injury | Tendinopatia Achille da overuse |
| Achilles tendon rupture | Rottura del tendine di Achille |
| Achillodynia (Achilles tendinitis) | Tendinopatia achillea (achillodinia) |
| Achlorhydria | Acloridria |
| Achondroplasia | Acondroplasia |
| Acidosis | Acidosi |
| Acne | Acne |
| Acne vulgaris | Acne volgare (acne) |
| Acoustic neuroma | Neuroma dell'acustico |
| Acrocyanosis | Acrocianosi |
| Acromegaly | Acromegalia |
| Acrophobia (fear of heights) | Acrofobia (paura dei luoghi elevati) |
| Actinic keratosis | Cheratosi solare |
| Actinomycosis | Actinomicosi |
| Acute abdomen | Addome acuto |
| Acute appendicitis | Appendicite acuta |
| Acute gastric dilatation | Dilatazione gastrica acuta |
| Acute kidney failure | Insufficienza renale acuta |
| Acute lymphoblastic leukemia | Leucemia acuta linfoblastica |
| Acute myeloid leukemia (AML) | Leucemia mieloide acuta |
| Acute pain | Dolore acuto |
| Acute pulmonary heart | Cuore polmonare acuto |
| Addiction | Dipendenza |
| Addison's disease | Morbo di Addison |
| Adenocarcinoma | Adenocarcinoma |
| Adenoma | Adenoma |
| Adenopathy | Adenopatia |
| African trypanosomiasis (sleeping sickness) | Tripanosomiasi africana (malattia del sonno) |
| Age-related hearing loss (presbycusis) | Perdita dell'udito dovuta all'avanzamento dell'età (presbiacusia) |

| | |
|---|---|
| Age-related long-sightedness (presbyopia) | Presbiopia (presbitismo) |
| Agenesis (absence of an organ) | Agenesia (mancanza di un organo) |
| Agnail (hangnail) | Pipita |
| Agranulocytosis | Agranulocitosi |
| AIDS (acquired immune deficiency syndrome) | SIDA (sindrome da ImmunoDeficienza Acquisita, AIDS) |
| Air embolism (gas embolism) | Embolia gassosa |
| Albinism | Albinismo |
| Albuminuria | Albuminuria |
| Alcohol poisoning | Avvelenamento da alcool |
| Alcoholic cardiomyopathy | Miocardiopatia alcolica |
| Alcoholic cirrhosis | Cirrosi alcolica |
| Alcoholism | Alcolismo |
| Aldosteronism (hyperaldosteronism) | Iperaldosteronismo |
| Algodystrophy | Algodistrofia |
| Alkali poisoning | Avvelenamento da alcali |
| Alkalosis | Alcalosi |
| Allergic contact dermatitis | Dermatite allergica |
| Allergic conjunctivitis | Congiuntivite allergica |
| Allergic rhinitis | Rinite allergica |
| Allergy | Allergia |
| Alopecia | Alopecia |
| Alopecia areata | Alopecia areata |
| Alopecia universalis | Alopecia universale |
| Altitude sickness (acute mountain sickness) | Mal di montagna |
| Alzheimer's diesase | Morbo di Alzheimer |
| Amebiasis (amebic dysentery) | Amebiasi |
| Amnesia | Amnesia |
| Amputation | Amputazione |
| Amyloidosis | Amiloidosi |
| Amyotrophic lateral sclerosis | Sclerosi laterale amiotrofica |
| Anal abscess | Ascesso anale |
| Anal atresia | Atresia anale |
| Anal bleeding | Perdita di sangue dall'ano (rettoragia, proctorragia) |
| Anal fissure | Fissura anale |
| Anal fistula | Fistola anale |
| Analgesia (loss of pain sensation) | Analgesia |
| Anaphylactic shock | Anafilassi |
| Anaplastic carcinoma | Carcinoma anaplastico |
| Ancylostomiasis | Anchilostomiasi |
| Androblastoma (Sertoli-Leydig cell tumor) | Androblastoma |
| Anemia | Anemia |
| Anemia of chronic disease | Anemia da malattia cronica |
| Anencephaly | Anencefalia |
| Aneurysm (aneurism) | Aneurisma |
| Aneurysm rupture | Rottura di aneurisma |
| Angina | Angina |
| Angina pectoris | Angina pectoris |
| Angioedema (angioneurotic edema) | Angioedema (edema di Quincke, edema angioneurotico) |
| Angioma | Angioma |
| Angiosarcoma | Angiosarcoma |
| Anisakiasis | Anisakidosi |
| Ankle arthrosis | Artrosi di caviglia |
| Ankle distortion | Distorsione alla caviglia |
| Ankle impingement syndrome | Sindrome da impingement della caviglia |
| Ankylosing spondylitis (Bechterew's syndrome) | Spondilite anchilosante |
| Ankylosis (joint stiffness) | Anchilosi |
| Anorexia | Anoressia |
| Ant sting | Puntura di formiche |
| Anterior cruciate ligament rupture (ACL rupture) | Rottura del legamento crociato anteriore del ginocchio |
| Anthracosis | Antracosi |
| Anthrax | Antrace |
| Anuria (passage of urine < 100 ml in 24 hours) | Anuria (produzione di urina < 100 ml nelle 24 ore) |
| Anxiety | Ansia (ansietà) |
| Aortic aneurysm | Aneurisma aortico |
| Aortic dissection | Dissecazione aortica |
| Aortic valve stenosis | Stenosi aortica |
| Aortoiliac occlusive disease (Leriche's syndrome) | Sindrome di Leriche |
| Aphtha (mouth ulcer) | Afta (ulcera all'interno della cavità orale) |
| Aplasia | Aplasia |
| Aplastic anemia | Anemia aplastica |
| Apoplexy | Apoplessia |
| Appetite | Appetito |
| Appetite changes | Cambiamenti nell'appetito |
| Aquaphobia | Idrofobia |
| Arrhythmia | Aritmia |
| Arrhythmogenic right ventricular dysplasia | Displasia ventricolare destra aritmogena |
| Arsenic poisoning | Avvelenamento da arsenico |

| | |
|---|---|
| Arterial bleeding | Emorragia arteriosa |
| Arterial embolism | Embolia dell'arteria |
| Arteriosclerosis | Arteriosclerosi |
| Arthrogryposis | Artrogriposi |
| Arthropathy | Artropatia |
| Arthrosis (osteoarthritis, degenerative arthritis) | Artrosi |
| Asbestos poisoning | Avvelenamento da amianto |
| Asbestosis | Asbestosi |
| Ascaridosis | Ascaridiasi |
| Ascites | Ascite |
| Aspergilloma (mycetoma, fungus ball) | Aspergilloma (micetoma) |
| Aspergillosis | Aspergillosi |
| Asphyxia | Asfissia |
| Asthma | Asma |
| Astigmatism | Astigmatismo |
| Astrocytoma | Astrocitoma |
| Atherosclerosis | Aterosclerosi |
| Athetosis | Atetosi |
| Athlete's foot (tinea pedis) | Piede d'atleta (tinea pedis) |
| Athlete's heart (cardiac hypertrophy) | Cuore dell'atleta (ipertrofia cardiaca da sport) |
| Atony (atonia) | Atonia muscolare |
| Atopic dermatitis | Neurodermite (dermatite atopica) |
| Atrial fibrillation | Fibrillazione atriale |
| Atrial septal defect | Difetto del setto interatriale |
| Atrioventricular block (AV block) | Blocco atrioventricolare |
| Atrophy | Atrofia |
| Attention deficit disorder | Disturbo della concentrazione |
| Atypical pneumonia | Polmonite atipica |
| Autism | Autismo |
| Autoimmune disease | Malattia autoimmunitaria |
| Aviophobia (fear of flying) | Aviofobia (paura di volare) |
| Avitaminosis | Avitaminosi |
| Baby colic | Coliche del neonato |
| Back pain (dorsalgia) | Mal di schiena (dorsopatia) |
| Bacteremia | Batteriemia |
| Bacterial conjunctivitis | Congiuntivite batterica |
| Bacterial endocarditis | Endocardite batterica |
| Bacterial infection | Infezione batterica |
| Bacterial pneumonia | Polmonite batterica |
| Bacterial vaginosis | Infezione della vagina batterica (vaginosi) |
| Bacteriuria | Batteriuria |
| Bad breath (halitosis) | Odore sgradevole dell'alito (alitosi, bromopnea) |
| Balance disorder | Disturbo dell'equilibrio |
| Ball-shaped aneurysm of the brain artery | Aneurisma cerebrale sferica |
| Barotrauma | Barotrauma |
| Bartonellosis | Bartonellosi |
| Basal cell carcinoma | Basalioma (carcinoma basocellulare) |
| Base of skull fracture (basal skull fracture) | Frattura della base del cranio |
| Basedow Graves disease | Morbo di Basedow-Graves |
| Basophilia | Basofilia |
| Bedsore (decubitus ulcer) | Piaga da decubito (decubito) |
| Behavioral disorder | Disturbo dell'umore |
| Behçet's disease | Sindrome di Behçet |
| Bell's palsy | Paralisi di Bell |
| Bell's phenomenon | Fenomeno di Bell |
| Benign positional vertigo | Cupololitiasi (canalolitiasi) |
| Benign prostatic hyperthroph | Ipertrofia prostatica benigna |
| Benign tumor | Tumore benigno |
| Bile duct atresia | Atresia biliare |
| Biliary cirrhosis | Cirrosi biliare |
| Biliary colic | Colica biliare |
| Biot's respiration | Respiro di Biot |
| Bipolar disorder (manic-depressive psychosis) | Psicosi maniaco-depressiva |
| Bird flu (influenza virus A subtype H5N1) | Influenza aviaria H5N1 |
| Birthmark (nevus) | Voglia (neo, nevo) |
| Bite | Morsicatura |
| Bite by rabies infected animal | Morsicatura di animale rabbioso |
| Bite wound | Ferita da morso |
| Black stool (melena) | Feci picee (melena) |
| Black widow bite | Morso della vedova nera |
| Bladder stone (urolithiasis) | Calcolo urinario (urolitiasi) |
| Blast-syndrome | Lesioni da scoppio (blast-syndrome) |
| Blastoma | Blastoma |
| Blastomycosis | Blastomicosi |
| Bleeding (haemorrhage) | Emorragia |
| Bleeding into joint space (hemarthrosis) | Emartro |
| Bleeding into the fallopian tube (hematosalpinx) | Flusso di sangue nella tuba di Falloppio |

| | |
|---|---|
| Blepharitis | Blefarite |
| Blindness | Cecità |
| Blister | Vescichetta (bolla) |
| Blister (corn) | Callo (vescica, bolla) |
| Bloating and gases (flatulence) | Gonfiezza e venti (flatulenza) |
| Blood clot (thrombus) | Trombo |
| Blood in cerebrospinal fluid | Sangue al liquido cerebrospinale |
| Blood in sputum (hemoptysis) | Sangue nello sputo (emottisi) |
| Blood in stool (hematochezia) | Sangue nelle feci (ematochezia) |
| Blood in urine (hematuria) | Ematuria |
| Blood pressure fall | Abbassamento della pressione del sangue |
| Blood vessel diseases | Malattie dei vasi sanguigni |
| Blount's disease | Sindrome di Blount |
| Bone bending (bone torsion) | Torsione dell'osso |
| Bone tuberculosis | Tubercolosi delle ossa |
| Borderline personality disorder | Disturbo borderline di personalità |
| Bornholm disease (epidemic myalgia) | Malattia di Bornholm (mialgia epidemica) |
| Borreliosis | Borreliosi |
| Botryoid sarcoma | Sarcoma botrioide |
| Botulism | Botulismo |
| Bouchard's nodes | Noduli di Bouchard |
| Bow legs (genu varum) | Ginocchio varo (genu varum) |
| Bowen's disease (squamous cell carcinoma in situ) | Morbo di Bowen |
| Brachial syndrome | Brachialgia |
| Brain abscess | Ascesso cerebrale |
| Brain compression | Compressione cerebrale |
| Brain concussion | Commozione cerebrale |
| Brain development anomaly | Anomalia di sviluppo del sistema nervoso |
| Brain laceration | Lacerazione cerebrale |
| Breast cancer | Cancro della mammella |
| Breast carcinoma | Carcinoma mammario |
| Breast pain (mastalgia) | Dolore al seno (mastalgia) |
| Breathing difficulty | Respirazione difficoltosa |
| Breathing sound due to blockage in the airway (stridor) | Rumore durante la respirazione (stridore) |
| Brenner tumour | Tumore di Brenner |
| Brill's disease | Malattia di Brill-Zinsser |
| Brodie abscess | Ascesso di Brodie |
| Broken ankle (ankle fracture) | Frattura della caviglia |
| Broken big toe (fractured hallux) | Frattura dell'alluce |
| Broken bone (bone fracture) | Frattura |
| Broken collar bone (clavicle fracture) | Frattura della clavicola |
| Broken elbow (olecranon fracture) | Frattura dell'olecrano |
| Broken fibula (fibula fracture) | Frattura della fibula |
| Broken finger (finger fracture) | Frattura della falange del dito |
| Broken foot (metatarsal fracture) | Frattura del metatarso |
| Broken forearm (fractured ulna and radius) | Frattura di radio e ulna |
| Broken heel bone (calcaneus fracture) | Frattura del calcagno |
| Broken knee cap (patellar fracture) | Frattura della rotula |
| Broken lower leg bones (fractured tibia and fibula) | Frattura di tibia e perone |
| Broken navicular bone (navicular fracture) | Frattura dell'osso navicolare |
| Broken pelvis (pelvis fracture) | Frattura del bacino |
| Broken rib (rib fracture) | Frattura della costola |
| Broken shinbone (tibia fracture) | Frattura della tibia |
| Broken shoulder blade (scapula fracture) | Frattura della scapola |
| Broken thighbone (femur fracture) | Frattura del femore |
| Broken ulna (ulna fracture) | Frattura dell'ulna |
| Broken upper arm (humerus fracture) | Frattura dell'omero |
| Broken vertebral body (vertebral corpus fracture) | Frattura del corpo vertebrale |
| Bronchial carcinoid | Carcinoide bronchiale |
| Bronchial carcinoma | Carcinoma bronchiale |
| Bronchiectasis | Bronchiectasia |
| Bronchopleural fistula | Fistola broncopleurica |
| Bronchopneumonia | Broncopolmonite |
| Bronchospasm | Broncospasmo |
| Brown urine | Urina marrone |

| | |
|---|---|
| Brucellosis | Brucellosi |
| Bruise (ecchymosis) | Ammaccatura (ecchimosi) |
| Buerger's disease (thromboangiitis obliterans) | Morbo di Buerger |
| Bulging eyes (exophthalmos) | Esoftalmo |
| Bulimia | Bulimia |
| Bundle branch block | Blocco di branca |
| Bunion | Alluce valgo |
| Burn | Ustione |
| Burning sensation | Sensazione bruciante |
| Burping (belching) | Eruttazione |
| Byssinosis (Monday fever) | Bissinosi |
| Cachexia | Cachessia |
| Cadmium poisoning | Avvelenamento da cadmio |
| Calcification | Calcificazione |
| Callosity (thickening) | Callosità (callo) |
| Candidiasis (thrush) | Candidosi (candidiasi) |
| Capillary hemangioma (infantile hemangioma, strawberry hemangioma) | Emangioma capillare |
| Carbon monoxide poisoning | Avvelenamento da monossido di carbonio |
| Carbuncle | Carbonchio (pustola) |
| Carcinoid | Carcinoide |
| Carcinoid syndrome | Sindrome da carcinoide |
| Carcinoma | Carcinoma |
| Carcinosis | Carcinosi (carcinomatosi, cancerosi) |
| Cardiac arrest (cardiopulmonary arrest) | Arresto cardiaco |
| Cardiac arrhythmia | Aritmia cardiaca |
| Cardiac asthma (paroxysmal nocturnal dyspnea) | Dispnea parossistica notturna |
| Cardiac decompensation | Decompensazione cardiaca |
| Cardiogenic shock | Shock cardiogeno |
| Cardiomyopathy | Cardiomiopatia |
| Cardiotoxicity | Cardiomiopatia tossica |
| Carpal tunnel syndrome | Sindrome del tunnel carpale |
| Cat bite | Morsicatura di gatto |
| Cat cry syndrome (5p minus syndrome, Lejeune's syndrome) | Sindrome del grido di gatto |
| Catalepsy | Catalessia |
| Cataplexy | Cataplessia |
| Cataract | Cataratta |
| Catarrh | Catarro |
| Cavernous hemangioma | Emangioma cavernoso |
| Cellulitis | Cellulite |
| Cephalocele | Cefalocèle |
| Cercaria | Cercaria |
| Cerebral aneurysm | Aneurisma cerebrale |
| Cerebral contusion | Contusione cerebrale |
| Cerebral edema | Edema cerebrale |
| Cerebral palsy | Paralisi cerebrale infantile |
| Cerebrovascular anomaly | Anomalia cerebrovascolare |
| Cervical cancer | Cancro della cervice uterina |
| Cervical carcinoma | Carcinoma della cervice uterina |
| Cervical dysplasia | Displasia cervicale |
| Cervical erosion | Erosione cervicale |
| Cervical polyp | Polipo cervicale |
| Cervical rib | Costa cervicale |
| Cervicobrachial syndrome | Sindrome cervicobrachiale (sindrome spalla-mano) |
| Cervicocephal syndrome | Sindrome cervicale |
| Chagas disease (American trypanosomiasis) | Malattia di Chagas |
| Chalicosis | Calicosi |
| Chancre | Sifiloma |
| Chancroid (soft chancre) | Ulcera venerea (cancroide) |
| Changes in consciousness | Alterazione della conoscenza |
| Changes in moles | Cambiamenti di nevi |
| Changes in mucous membrane | Cambiamenti della mucosa |
| Changes in olfactory sensation | Cambiamenti delle sensazoni olfattive |
| Changes in shape of bones | Cambiamenti nella forma delle ossa |
| Changes in tactile sensation | Cambiamenti della sensazione tattile |
| Changes in taste sensation | Cambiamenti nelle sensazioni del gusto |
| Charcot-Marie-Tooth disease | Malattia di Charcot-Marie-Tooth |
| Chemical conjunctivitis | Congiuntivite irritativa da agenti chimici |
| Chemical injuries | Ferita chimica |

| | |
|---|---|
| Chemical warfare poisoning | Avvelenamento da armi chimiche |
| Chest pain | Dolore toracico |
| Chicken-pox | Varicella |
| Chikungunya | Chikungunya |
| Chilblain (perniosis) | Perniosi |
| Childhood infectious diseases | Malattie infettive dei bambini |
| Chlamydia infection | Infezione da clamidia |
| Choking (suffocation) | Soffocamento (soffocazione, asfissia) |
| Cholangiocellular carcinoma | Colangiocarcinoma (carcinoma colangiocellulare) |
| Cholera | Colera |
| Chondroblastoma | Condroblastoma |
| Chondroma | Condroma |
| Chondromalacia patellae (runner's knee, patello-femoral pain syndrome) | Sindrome del dolore patello-femorale (ginocchio del corridoro) |
| Chondromyxoid fibroma | Fibroma condromixoide |
| Chondrosarcoma | Condrosarcoma |
| Choreoathetosis | Coreoatetosi |
| Choriocarcinoma | Coriocarcinoma |
| Chromoblastomycosis (chromomycosis, Pedroso's disease) | Cromomicosi (cromoblastomicosi) |
| Chronic cerebrospinal venous insufficiency | Insufficienza venosa cronica cerebrospinale |
| Chronic fatigue syndrome | Sindrome da fatica cronica |
| Chronic lymphocytic leukemia | Leucemia linfatica cronica |
| Chronic myeloid leukemia | Leucemia mieloide cronica |
| Chronic obstructive pulmonary disease | Bronchite cronica |
| Chronic pain | Dolore cronico |
| Chronic paroxysmal hemicrania (Sjaastad syndrome) | Emicrania cronica parossistica |
| Chronic renal failure | Insufficienza renale cronica |
| Chylothorax | Chilotorace |
| Claustrophobia (fear of closed space) | Claustrofobia (paura di luoghi chiusi) |
| Cleft lip and palate | Labbro leporino |
| Clonorchiasis | Clonorchiasi |
| Clostridium perfringens toxic infection | Tossinfezione da Clostridium perfringens |
| Club foot (talipes equinovarus) | Piede equino (talipes equinovarus) |
| Cluster headache | Cefalea a grappolo |
| Coagulation factor deficiency | Carenza di fattore di coagulazione |
| Coarctation of the aorta | Coartazione dell'aorta |
| Coccidioidomycosis (San Joaquin Valley fever) | Coccidiomicosi |
| Coccygodynia | Coccigodinia |
| Coeliac disease (celiac disease) | Celiachia (malattia caliaca) |
| Colic | Colica |
| Collapse | Collasso |
| Colon diverticulum | Diverticolo del colon |
| Colon polyp | Polipo del colon |
| Colorado tick fever (mountain tick fever) | Febbre da zecca del Colorado |
| Coma | Coma |
| Comminuted fracture | Frattura comminuta |
| Common cold | Infreddatura (raffreddore) |
| Compartment syndrome | Sindrome compartimentale |
| Confusion | Confusione (disordine) |
| Congenital aneurysm of arteries at the base of the brain | Aneurisma arteriosa congenita alla base dell'encefalo |
| Congenital dysplasia of the hip (congenital hip dislocation) | Lussazione congenita dell'anca (displasia dell'anca) |
| Congenital heart defect | Difetto cardiaco congenito |
| Congenital heart disease (congenital cardiopathy) | Cardiopatia congenita |
| Congenital pyloric stenosis | Stenosi pilorica congenita |
| Conjunctival foreign body | Congiuntivite irritativa da corpi estranei |
| Constipation (obstipation) | Stitichezza (costipazione) |
| Contact dermatitis | Dermatite da contatto |
| Contracture | Contrattura |
| Contusion | Contusione |
| Convulsions | Convulsioni |
| Coronary disease | Coronaropatia |
| Cough | Tosse |

| | |
|---|---|
| Cradle cap (infantile seborrhoeic dermatitis) | Dermatite seborroica infantile |
| Cranial neuralgia | Nevralgia del nervo cranico |
| Crepitation | Crepitazione |
| Creutzfeldt-Jakob disease (so called "mad cow disease") | Malattia di Creutzfeldt-Jakob (cosiddetta "malattia della mucca pazza") |
| Crimean-Congo hemorrhagic fever | Febbre emorragica Crimean-Congo |
| Crohn's disease | Malattia di Crohn |
| Crotch itch (tinea cruris) | Tinea cruris |
| Croup (acute obstructive laryngitis) | Croup (laringite acuta ostruttiva) |
| Crush-syndrome | Sindrome da schiacciamento |
| Crust (scab) | Crosta (escara) |
| Cryptococcosis | Criptococcosi |
| Cryptogenic cirrhosis | Cirrosi criptogenica |
| Cryptorchidism | Criptorchidismo |
| Cushing's syndrome (hypercorticism) | Sindrome di Cushing (ipercortisolismo) |
| Cut wound | Ferita da taglio |
| Cutaneous leishmaniasis (Oriental sore) | Leishmaniosi cutanea |
| Cyanide poisoning | Avvelenamento da cianuro |
| Cyanosis | Cianosi |
| Cyst | Cisti (ciste) |
| Cystadenocarcinoma | Cistadenocarcinoma |
| Cystadenofibroma | Cistadenofibroma |
| Cystadenoma | Cistadenoma |
| Cystic fibrosis | Fibrosi cistica |
| Cysticercosis | Cisticercosi |
| Cystoma | Cistoma |
| Daltonism | Daltonismo |
| Dancer's foot (pes equinus) | Piede equino |
| Dancer's tendinitis (flexor hallucis tendinitis) | Tendinite del flessore lungo dell'alluce |
| Dandruff | Forfora |
| Day blindness (hemeralopia) | Emeralopia |
| Deafness | Sordità |
| Death | Morte |
| Decompression sickness (diver's disease, caisson disease) | Malattia di decompressione (sindrome di Caisson) |
| Decreased body temperature (hypothermia) | Bassa temperatura corporea (ipotermia) |
| Decreased production of urine (oliguria) | Diminuita escrezione urinaria (oliguria) |
| Dehydration | Disidratazione |
| Delayed puberty | Pubertà tardiva |
| Delirium | Delirio |
| Dementia | Demenza |
| Demineralization | Demineralizzazione |
| Dengue fever | Dengue |
| Dental caries | Carie dentaria |
| Dental plaque (dental tartar) | Placca (tartaro) |
| Depression | Depressione |
| DeQuervain syndrome | Sindrome di De Quervain |
| Dermatitis herpetiformis (Duhring's disease) | Dermatite erpetiforme di Duhring |
| Dermatomycosis | Dermatomicosi |
| Dermatomyositis | Dermatomiosite |
| Dermoid cyst | Cisti dermoide |
| Development anomalies | Anomalie di sviluppo |
| Diabetes | Diabete |
| Diabetes insipidus | Diabete insipido |
| Diabetes mellitus | Diabete mellito |
| Diabetes mellitus type 1 | Diabete mellito di tipo 1 |
| Diabetes mellitus type 2 | Diabete mellito di tipo 2 |
| Diabetic coma | Coma diabetico |
| Diabetic ketoacidosis | Chetoacidosi diabetica |
| Diabetic nephropathy | Nefropatia diabetica |
| Diabetic neuropathy | Neuropatia diabetica |
| Diabetic retinopathy | Retinopatia diabetica |
| Diaphragmatic hernia | Ernia diaframmatica |
| Diaphyseal humeral fracture | Frattura diafisaria dell'omero |
| Diaphyseal tightbone fracture | Frattura della diafisi femorale |
| Diarrhea | Diarrea |
| Difficult defecation (tenesmus) | Difficoltà a defecare (tenesmo) |
| Difficult urination (dysuria) | Emissione di urine con difficoltà (disuria) |
| Difficult swallowing (dysphagia) | Difficoltà a deglutire (disfagia) |
| Dilated cardiomyopathy | Cardiomiopatia dilatativa |
| Diphtheria | Difterite |
| Discarthrosis (degenerative disc disease) | Discartrosi (discopatia degenerativa) |
| Discharge | Fuoriuscita (scolo) |
| Diseases of the aorta | Malattie dell'aorta |

| | |
|---|---|
| Dislocated ankle joint | Lussazione della caviglia |
| Dislocated fragments | Dislocazione dei frammenti |
| Dislocated shoulder | Lussazione della spalla |
| Dislocation (luxation) | Lussazione |
| Dislocation of a hip | Lussazione dell'anca |
| Disorientation | Disorientamento |
| Disseminated intravascular coagulation | Coagulazione intravascolare disseminata |
| Distal radial fracture | Frattura di Pouteau-Colles (frattura delle metafisi radiali distali) |
| Diverticulitis | Diverticolite |
| Diverticulosis | Diverticolosi |
| Diverticulum | Diverticolo |
| Dizziness (vertigo) | Capogiro (vertigine) |
| Dog bite | Morsicatura di cane |
| Double vision (diplopia) | Visione doppia (diplopia) |
| Down syndrome | Sindrome di Down |
| Dracunculiasis | Dracunculiasi |
| Drooling (ptyalism, sialorrhea, slobbering) | Sbavando (ptialismo, scialorrea) |
| Drooping of the upper eyelid (blepharoptosis) | Spostamento della palpebra (palpebra calante, blefaroptosi) |
| Drowning | Affogamento |
| Drug addiction | Tossicodipendenza (tossicomania) |
| Drug allergy | Allergia a farmaci |
| Drug overdose | Overdose di droga |
| Dry cough | Tosse secca |
| Dry eyes (keratoconjuctivitis sicca) | Occhi secchi (xeroftalmia) |
| Dry gangrene | Gangrena secca |
| Dry mouth (xerostomia) | Scarsa secrezione salivare (xerostomia) |
| Duchenne muscular dystrophy | Distrofia di Duchenne |
| Ductus arteriosus (ductus Botalli shunt) | Dotto arterioso di Botallo |
| Dull pain | Dolore ottuso |
| Dullness in limbs | Ottusità alle estremità |
| Duodenal atresia | Atresia duodenale |
| Duodenal diverticulum | Diverticolo duodenale |
| Duodenal ulcer | Ulcera duodenale |
| Dupuytren's contracture | Malattia di Dupuytren |
| Dust allergy | Allergia a polvere |
| Dwarfism (nanism) | Nanismo |
| Dyschondroplasia | Discondroplasia |
| Dysentery (flux) | Dissenteria |
| Dysgerminoma | Disgerminoma |
| Dyshidrosis | Disidrosi |
| Dyslexia | Dislessia |
| Dyspepsia (upset stomach) | Dispepsia |
| Dystonia | Distonia |
| Dystrophy | Distrofia |
| Ear bleeding | Fuoriuscita di sangue dall'orecchio (otorragia) |
| Ear pain (otalgia) | Dolore auricolare (otalgia) |
| Early symptom (prodrome) | Sindrome prodromica |
| Eating disorder | Disturbo del comportamento alimentare |
| Ebola hemorrhagic fever | Ebola |
| Echinococcosis (hydatid disease) | Echinococcosi (idatidosi) |
| Echolalia | Ecolalia |
| Echopraxia (involuntary repetition of the observed movements of another person) | Ecoprassia (imitazione spontanea di movimenti osservati) |
| Ectopic pregnancy (extrauterine pregnancy) | Gravidanza ectopica |
| Eczema | Eczema |
| Edema | Edema |
| Edwards syndrome (trisomy 18) | Sindrome di Edwards |
| Eisenmenger's syndrome | Sindrome di Eisenmenger |
| Elbow arthrosis | Artrosi di gomito |
| Elbow dislocation (luxation of the elbow) | Lussazione del gomito |
| Electric shock burn | Ustione da corrente elettrica |
| Electrical injuries (electric shock) | Folgorazione (elettrocuzione) |
| Electromagnetic hypersensitivity | Elettrosensibilità |
| Elephantiasis (lymphedema) | Elefantiasi |
| Elevated body temperature | Temperatura corporea elevata |
| Embolism | Embolismo (embolia) |
| Embryonal carcinoma | Carcinoma embrionale |
| Emphysema | Enfisema |
| Empyema | Empiema |
| Encephalocele | Encefalocele |
| Encephalopathy | Encefalopatia |
| Enchondroma | Encondroma |
| Encopresis | Enconpresi |

| | |
|---|---|
| Endocardial fibroelastosis | Fibroelastosi endocardica |
| Endometrial carcinoma | Carcinoma endometriale |
| Endometrial hyperplasia | Iperplasia endometriale |
| Endometrial polyp (uterine polyp) | Polipo endometriale |
| Endometriosis | Endometriosi |
| Endotoxic shock | Shock endotossico |
| Enlarged liver (hepatomegaly) | Aumento di volume del fegato (epatomegalia) |
| Enlarged lymph nodes (lymphadenopathy) | Ingrossamento dei linfonodi (linfoadenopatia) |
| Enlarged pupils | Pupille dilatate |
| Enlarged tongue (macroglossia) | Eccessiva crescita della lingua (macroglossia) |
| Enthesopathy | Entesopatia |
| Eosinophilia | Eosinofilia |
| Ependymoma | Ependimoma |
| Epicondylar elbow fracture | Frattura dell'epicondilo omerale |
| Epidemic typhus (louse-borne typhus) | Tifo esantematico (tifo epidemico) |
| Epidural bleeding | Emorragia epidurale |
| Epidural hematoma | Ematoma epidurale |
| Epigastric pain | Gastralgia |
| Epilepsy | Epilessia |
| Epiphyseolysis capitis femoris | Epifisiolisi della testa femorale |
| Epispadias | Epispadia |
| Epithelial carcinoma | Carcinoma epiteliale |
| Erysipelas (Ignis sacer, St. Anthony's fire) | Erisipela |
| Erysipeloid | Erisipeloide |
| Erythromelalgia (acromelalgia) | Eritromelalgia |
| Erythroplakia (erythroplasia) | Eritroplachia (eritroplasia) |
| Erythroplasia of Queyrat | Eritroplasia di Queyrat |
| Esophageal atresia | Atresia esofagea |
| Esophageal stenosis | Stenosi esofagea |
| Esophageal varices | Varici esofagee |
| Essential hypertension | Ipertensione arteriosa essenziale |
| Estrogen deficiency | Carenza di estrogeno |
| Ewing's sarcoma | Sarcoma di Ewing |
| Exanthem | Esantema |
| Exanthema subitum (roseola infantum, sixth disease) | Sesta malattia (roseola infantum, esantema subitum) |
| Exasperation | Esasperazione (irritazione) |
| Excessive hunger (polyphagia) | Aumento incontrollato dell'appetito (polifagia) |
| Excessive secretion of saliva (hypersalivation) | Produzione di saliva eccessiva (ipersalivazione) |
| Excessive sweating (hyperhidrosis) | Aumento della sudorazione (iperidrosi) |
| Exostosis | Esostosi |
| Expectoration of blood (hemoptysis) | Espettorazione di sangue (emottisi) |
| Explosive wound | Ferita esplosiva |
| Expulsion of undigested food from stomack to the mouth (regurgitation) | Risalita di alimenti dallo stomaco alla bocca (rigurgito) |
| Extensor tendinitis (inflammation of the extensor tendons of the toes) | Tendinite dei estensori delle dita del piede |
| External abdominal wall hernia | Ernia esterna addominale |
| External bleeding | Emorragia esterna |
| Extrajoint rheumatism | Reumatismo extra-articolare |
| Facial spasm | Spasmo facciale |
| Familial Mediterranean fever | Febbre mediterranea familiare |
| Farmer's lung | Febbre da fieno |
| Farsightedness (hyperopia) | Ipermetropia |
| Fat embolism | Embolia adiposa |
| Fatigue (exhaustion, lethargy) | Stanchezza (fatica, astenia) |
| Fatty liver metamorphosis | Metamorfosi grassa del fegato |
| Favus | Tinea favosa |
| Feather allergy | Allergia alle piume |
| Febrile convulsions | Convulsioni febbrili |
| Femoral neck fracture | Frattura del collo del femore |
| Fetal alcohol syndrome | Sindrome alcolica fetale |
| Fever | Febbre |
| Fibrinoid necrosis | Necrosi fibrinoide |
| Fibroadenoma | Fibroadenoma |
| Fibrocystic breast disease | Mastopatia fibrocistica |
| Fibroma | Fibroma |
| Fibromyalgia | Fibromialgia |
| Fibrosarcoma (fibroblastic sarcoma) | Fibrosarcoma |
| Fibrosis | Fibrosi |
| Fibrous dysplasia | Displasia fibrosa |
| Fibrous histiocytoma | Fibroistiocitoma benigno |
| Filariasis | Filariasi |

| | |
|---|---|
| Finger clubbing (digital clubbing) | Dita ippocratiche (dita a bacchetta di tamburo) |
| First menstrual cycle (menarche) | Primo flusso mestruale (menarca) |
| Fish poisoning | Avvelenamento da pesci |
| Fistula | Fistola |
| Flaccid muscle (untoned muscle) | Muscolo flaccido |
| Flat foot (pes planus) | Piede piatto (pes planus) |
| Floating kidney (nephroptosis, renal ptosis) | Spostamento del rene (ptosi renale, nefroptosi) |
| Floppy infant syndrome | Sindrome del bambino flaccido |
| Flu (influenza) | Influenza |
| Foamy sputum | Sputo schiumoso |
| Folliculitis | Follicolite |
| Food allergy | Allergia alimentare |
| Food aversion | Ripugnanza al cibo |
| Food poisoning | Avvelenamento da cibo |
| Foot arthrosis | Artrosi al piede |
| Foot deformity | Difetto del piede |
| Forearm tendinitis | Tendinite dell'avambraccio |
| Foreign body in ear | Corpo estraneo nell'orecchio |
| Foreign body in nose | Corpo estraneo nel naso |
| Fournier gangrene | Gangrena di Fournier |
| Fracture with displacement | Frattura con dislocazione |
| Freiberg's disease | Malattia di Freiberg |
| Frequent urination | Urinazione frequente (pollachiuria) |
| Frequent urination at night (nocturia) | Urinazione notturna (nicturia) |
| Frigidity | Frigidità |
| Frostbite | Congelamento |
| Frozen shoulder (adhesive capsulitis of shoulder) | Capsulite adesiva |
| Fungal infection | Infezione fungina |
| Fungal osteomyelitis | Osteomielite fungale |
| Fur allergy | Allergia a pello di animali |
| Furuncle (boil) | Foruncolo |
| Gaining weight | Ingrossamento (divenire grosso) |
| Galactorrhea | Galattorrea |
| Gallbladder hydrops | Idrope della colecisti |
| Gallstone (cholelithiasis) | Calcolo biliare |
| Gambling addiction (ludomania) | Giocco d'azzardo patologico |
| Gangrene | Cancrena |
| Gas gangrene | Gangrene gassosa |
| Gas poisoning | Avvelenamento da gas |
| Gastric carcinoma | Carcinoma gastrico |
| Gastric ulcer | Ulcera gastrica |
| Gastroenteritis | Gastroenterite |
| Generalized edema (anasarca) | Edema diffuso (anasarca) |
| Genital herpes | Herpes genitalis |
| Genital wart | Condiloma |
| German measles (rubella) | Rosolia |
| Giant cell arteritis (temporal arteritis) | Arterite temporale (arterite di Horton) |
| Gigantism | Gigantismo |
| Gigantocellular tumor (osteoclastoma) | Osteoclastoma (tumore a cellule giganti) |
| Glanders | Morva umana |
| Glaucoma | Glaucoma |
| Glioblastoma | Glioblastoma |
| Glioma | Glioma |
| Gliosis | Gliosi |
| Glomerulonephritis | Glomerulonefrite |
| Glomus tumor (glomangioma) | Glomangioma (paraganglioma) |
| Glucose in urine (glycosuria) | Glicosuria (mellituria) |
| Gluten intolerance | Intolleranza al glutine |
| Goiter | Gozzo |
| Gonadoblastoma | Gonadoblastoma |
| Gonorrhea | Gonorrea (blenorragia) |
| Goodpasture's syndrome | Sindrome di Goodpasture |
| Gout (gouty arthritis) | Gotta |
| Granulocytosis | Granulocitosi |
| Granulomatous inflammation | Infiammazione granulomatosa |
| Granulosa cell tumor | Follicoloma |
| Green stool | Feci di colore verde |
| Greenstick fracture | Frattura a legno verde |
| Groin pain syndrome | Pubalgia dello sportivo |
| Guillain-Barré syndrome | Sindrome di Guillain-Barré |
| Gunshot wound | Ferita da arma da fuoco |
| Gymnastics lower back pain | Lombalgia dell'atleta |
| Gynecomastia | Ginecomastia |
| Haglund's disease | Malattia di Haglund (deformità di Haglund) |
| Hallucination | Allucinazione |
| Hand and finger joints dislocation | Lussazioni delle atricolazioni della mano e delle dita |

| | |
|---|---|
| Hand arthrosis | Artrosi della mano |
| Hand fibrositis | Fibrosite di mano |
| Hand tremor | Tremore delle mani |
| Hand-arm vibration syndrome (vibration white finger) | Sindrome da vibrazioni mano-braccio |
| Hard of hearing | Sordità parziale |
| Hashimoto's disease | Tiroidite di Hashimoto |
| Head and brain injuries | Lesioni della testa e del cervello |
| Headache | Mal di testa |
| Hearing disorder | Disturbo dell'udito |
| Hearing loss | Perdita di udito |
| Heart attack (myocardial infarction) | Infarto miocardico acuto |
| Heart disease (cardiopathy) | Malattia del cuore (cardiopatia) |
| Heart murmur | Soffio cardiaco |
| Heart valve diseases | Malattie delle valvole cardiache |
| Heartburn | Bruciore di stomaco (pirosi) |
| Heavy metal poisoning | Intossicazione da metalli pesanti |
| Heberden's nodes | Noduli di Heberden |
| Heel spur (calcaneal spur) | Spina nel calcagno (spina calcaneare) |
| Hemangioendothelioma | Emangioendotelioma |
| Hemangioma | Emangioma |
| Hematoma | Ematoma |
| Hemivertebrae | Emivertebra |
| Hemochromatosis | Emocromatosi |
| Hemoglobin in urine (hemoglobinuria) | Presenza di emoglobina nelle urine (emoglobinuria) |
| Hemolytic anemia | Anemia emolitica |
| Hemophilia | Emofilia |
| Hemophiliac arthropathy | Artropatia emofilica |
| Hemopneumothorax | Emopneumotorace |
| Hemorrhagic brain infarction | Ictus emorragico |
| Hemorrhagic fever with renal syndrome (Korean hemorrhagic fever) | Febbre emorragica con sindrome renale (febbre emorragica coreana) |
| Hemorrhoids | Emorroidi |
| Hemosiderosis | Emosiderosi |
| Hemothorax | Emotorace |
| Hepatic echinococcosis | Echinococcosi epatica |
| Hepatic tuberculosis | Tubercolosi epatica |
| Hepatitis A | Epatite virale A |
| Hepatitis B | Epatite virale B |
| Hepatitis C | Epatite virale C |
| Hepatitis D | Epatite virale D |
| Hepatitis E | Epatite virale E |
| Hepatocellular adenoma | Adenoma epatocellulare |
| Hepatocellular carcinoma | Carcinoma epatocellulare |
| Hepatorenal syndrome | Sindrome epato-renale |
| Hereditary ataxia | Atassia ereditaria |
| Hereditary multiple exostoses | Esostosi multipla ereditaria |
| Hermaphroditism | Ermafroditismo |
| Hernia | Ernia |
| Hernia sack | Sacco dell'ernia |
| Herpangina (mouth blisters) | Erpangina (faringite vescicolare) |
| Herpes simplex | Herpes simplex |
| Herpes zoster | Herpes zoster |
| Hiatus hernia | Ernia iatale |
| Hiccup | Singhiozzo |
| High arches (pes cavus) | Piede cavo (pes cavus) |
| High blood cholesterol (hypercholesterolemia) | Eccesso di colesterolo nel sangue (ipercolesterolemia) |
| High blood pressure (hypertension) | Ipertensione arteriosa sistemica |
| High blood sugar (hyperglicemia) | Eccesso di glucosio nel sangue (iperglicemia) |
| Hip arthrosis | Artrosi di anca |
| Hirschsprung's disease (congenital aganglionic megacolon) | Malattia di Hirschsprung (malattia di Mya) |
| Hirsutism | Irsutismo |
| Histoplasmosis (Darling's disease) | Istoplasmosi |
| Hives (urticaria) | Orticaria |
| Hoarseness | Raucedine |
| Hodgkin's disease | Linfoma di Hodgkin |
| Hoffa's disease | Sindrome di Hoffa |
| Horseshoe kidney (renal fusion) | Rene a ferro di cavallo (fusione renale) |
| Hot flushes | Vampata di calore |
| Human bite | Morsicatura di uomo |
| Human papilloma virus (HPV) infection | Infezione da Papilloma Virus Umano (HPV) |
| Humeral neck fracture | Frattura del collo dell'omero |
| Hunchback | Gibbo (gobba, gibbosità) |
| Hunger | Fame |
| Huntington's chorea (Huntington's disease) | Malattia di Huntington |

| | |
|---|---|
| Hyaline membrane disease (infant respiratory distress syndrome) | Sindrome da distress respiratorio del neonato (malattia da membrane ialine polmonari) |
| Hydremia | Idremia |
| Hydrocele | Idrocele |
| Hydrocephalus | Idrocefalo |
| Hydronephrosis | Idronefrosi |
| Hydrops | Idrope |
| Hydrothorax | Idrotorace |
| Hygroma | Igroma |
| Hyperactivity | Iperattività |
| Hypercalcemia | Ipercalcemia |
| Hyperinsulinism | Iperinsulinismo |
| Hyperkalemia | Iperkaliemia |
| Hyperparathyroidism | Iperparatiroidismo |
| Hyperpituitarism | Iperpituitarismo |
| Hyperthermia | Ipertermia |
| Hyperthropic osteoarthropaty (Pierre Marie-Bamberger syndrome) | Osteoartropatia ipertrofizzante (sindrome di Pierre Marie-Bamberger) |
| Hyperthyroidism | Ipertiroidismo |
| Hypertrophic cardiomyopathy | Cardiomiopatia ipertrofica |
| Hypertrophic pyloric stenosis | Stenosi ipertrofica del piloro |
| Hypertrophy | Ipertrofia |
| Hyperuricemia | Iperuricemia |
| Hyperventilation | Iperventilazione |
| Hypervitaminosis | Ipervitaminosi |
| Hypervolemia (increased level of fluid in the blood) | Ipervolemia (aumento del volume ematico circolante) |
| Hyphema | Ifema |
| Hypoalbuminemia | Ipoalbuminemia |
| Hypocalcemia | Ipocalcemia |
| Hypochondria | Ipocondria |
| Hypochromic anemia | Anemia ipocromica |
| Hypoglycemia | Ipoglicemia |
| Hypoinsulinism | Ipoinsulinemia |
| Hypokalemia | Ipokaliemia |
| Hypoparathyroidism | Ipoparatiroidismo |
| Hypopituitarism | Ipopituitarismo |
| Hypospadias | Ipospadia |
| Hypotension and syncope | Ipotensione e sincope |
| Hypothermia | Ipotermia |
| Hypothyroidism | Ipotiroidismo |
| Hypotonia | Ipotonia |
| Hypovolemic shock | Shock ipovolemico |
| Hypoxia | Ipossia |
| Hysteria | Isteria (isterismo) |
| Idiopathic pulmonary fibrosis | Fibrosi polmonare idiopatica |
| Ileus | Ileo |
| Iliotibial band friction syndrome | Sindrome della benderella ileotibiale |
| Imbecility | Imbecillità |
| Immunodeficiency | Immunodeficienza |
| Impacted cerumen | Tappo di cerume |
| Impetigo | Impetigine |
| Impotency | Impotenza |
| Inability to urinate | Mancata secrezione di urina |
| Incomplete fracture | Frattura incompleta (infrazione) |
| Incontinence | Incontinenza |
| Increased distance between two organs or parts of the body (hypertelorism) | Aumento della distanza fra due parti del corpo (ipertelorismo) |
| Increased hair loss | Aumento di perdita di capelli |
| Increased hairiness (hypertrichosis) | Aumento della pelosità (ipertricosi) |
| Increased sensitivity to stimuli of the senses (hyperesthesia) | Ippersensibilità ai normali stimoli esterni (iperestesia) |
| Increased thirst senasation (polydipsia) | Aumento del senso della sete (polidipsia) |
| Indigestion | Indigestione |
| Infarct | Infarto |
| Infected mosquito bite | Puntura di zanzara infetta |
| Infected tick bite | Morsicatura di zecca infetta |
| Infection | Infezione (malattia infettiva) |
| Infection of the bone or bone marrow (osteomyelitis) | Infezione dell'apparato osteo-articolare (osteomielite) |
| Infectious arthritis (septic arthritis) | Artrite settica |
| Infectious erythema (fifth disease) | Eritema infettivo (quinta malattia) |
| Infectious mononucleosis (Pfeiffer's disease, kissing disease, glandular fever) | Mononucleosi infettiva (malattia del bacio) |
| Infertility (sterility) | Sterilità (infecondità) |
| Infestation with head lice (pediculosis) | Infestazione da pidocchi (pediculosi) |
| Infestation with intestinal parasitic warms (helminthiasis) | Infestazione da vermi (elmintiasi) |
| Infestation with pubic lice (phthiriasis) | Infestazione da pidocchi del pube (ftiriasi) |
| Inflammation | Infiammazione (flogosi) |

| | |
|---|---|
| Inflammation of the appendix (appendicitis) | Infiammazione dell'appendice vermiforme (appendicite) |
| Inflammation of the arterial walls (arteritis) | Infiammazione delle arterie (arterite) |
| Inflammation of the brain (encephalitis) | Infiammazione del cervello (encefalite) |
| Inflammation of the breast (mastitis) | Infiammazione della mammella (mastite) |
| Inflammation of the bronchi (bronchitis) | Infiammazione dei bronchi (bronchite) |
| Inflammation of the bronchioles (bronchiolitis) | Infiammazione dei bronchioli (bronchiolite) |
| Inflammation of the conjunctiva (conjunctivitis) | Infiammazione della congiuntiva (congiuntivite) |
| Inflammation of the cornea (keratitis) | Infiammazione della cornea (cheratite) |
| Inflammation of the cornea and conjunctiva (kerato-conjunctivitis) | Infiammazione della cornea e della congiutiva (cherato-congiuntivite) |
| Inflammation of the endocardium (endocarditis) | Infiammazione dell'endocardio (endocardite) |
| Inflammation of the endometrium (endometritis) | Infiammazione dell'endometrio (endometrite) |
| Inflammation of entheses (enthesitis) | Infiammazione dell'inserzione di muscolo (entesite) |
| Inflammation of the epididymis (epididymitis) | Infiammazione dell'epididimo (epididimite) |
| Inflammation of the epiglottis (epiglottitis) | Infiammazione del'epiglottide (epiglottite) |
| Inflammation of the fascia (fasciitis) | Infiammazione della fascia (fascite) |
| Inflammation of the gall bladder (cholecystitis) | Infiammazione della colecisti (colecistite) |
| Inflammation of the glans penis (balanitis) | Infiammazione della testa del glande (balanite) |
| Inflammation of the gums (gingivitis) | Infiammazione dei tessuti gengivali (gengivite) |
| Inflammation of the heart muscle (myocarditis) | Infiammazione del miocardio (miocardite) |
| Inflammation of the inner ear (labyrinthitis) | Infiammazione di labirinto nell'orecchio interno (labirintite) |
| Inflammation of the joint (arthritis) | Infiammazione articolare (artrite) |
| Inflammation of the kidney (nephritis) | Infiammazione dei reni (nefrite) |
| Inflammation of the larynx (laryngitis) | Infiammazione della laringe (laringite) |
| Inflammation of the liver (hepatitis) | Infiammazione del fegato (epatite) |
| Inflammation of the lung (pneumonia) | Infiammazione dei polmoni (polmonite) |
| Inflammation of the lymph node (lymphadenitis) | Infiammazione delle ghiandole linfatiche (linfoadenite) |
| Inflammation of the meninges (meningitis) | Infiammazione delle meningi (meningite) |
| Inflammation of the middle layer of the eye (uveitis) | Infiammazione della tunica media dell'occhio (uveite) |
| Inflammation of the mouth mucous lining (stomatitis) | Infiammazione delle mucose della bocca (stomatite) |
| Inflammation of the muscles (myositis) | Infiammazione del tessuto muscolare (miosite) |
| Inflammation of the nerve (neuritis) | Infiammazione del nervo (neurite, nevrite) |
| Inflammation of the pancreas (pancreatitis) | Infiammazione del pancreas (pancreatite) |
| Inflammation of the parametrium (parametritis) | Infiammazione del parametrio (parametrite) |
| Inflammation of the paranasal sinuses (sinusitis) | Infiammazione dei seni paranasali (sinusite) |
| Inflammation of the pericardium (pericarditis) | Infiammazione del pericardio (pericardite) |
| Inflammation of the peritoneum (peritonitis) | Infiammazione dela sierosa peritoneale (peritonite) |
| Inflammation of the pleura (pleuritis) | Infiammazione della pleura (pleurite) |
| Inflammation of the prostate gland (prostatitis) | Infiammazione della ghiandola prostatica (prostatite) |
| Inflammation of the retina (retinitis) | Infiammazione della retina (retinite) |
| Inflammation of the salivary gland (sialadenitis) | Infiammazione delle ghiandole salivari (sialoadenite) |
| Inflammation of the skin (dermatitis) | Infiammazione della pelle (dermatite) |
| Inflammation of the stomach lining (gastritis) | Infiammazione della mucosa gastrica (gastrite) |
| Inflammation of the synovial fluid sac (bursitis) | Infiammazione della borsa sierosa di un'articolazione (borsite) |
| Inflammation of the synovial membrane (synovitis) | Infiammazione della membrana sinoviale (sinovite) |

| | |
|---|---|
| Inflammation of the synovium and tendon (tenosynovitis) | Infiammazione di tendine e di guaina tendinea (tenosinovite) |
| Inflammation of the tendon (tendinitis, tendonitis) | Infiammazione del tendine (tendinite) |
| Inflammation of the testes (orchitis) | Infiammazione dei testicoli (orchite) |
| Inflammation of the thymus (thymitis) | Infiammazione del timo |
| Inflammation of the thyroid gland (thyroiditis) | Infiammazione della tiroide (tiroidite) |
| Inflammation of the tonsils (tonsillitis) | Infiammazione delle tonsille (tonsillite) |
| Inflammation of the urethra (urethritis) | Infiammazione dell'uretra (uretrite) |
| Inflammation of the urinary bladder (cystitis) | Infiammazione della vescica urinaria (cistite) |
| Inflammation of the vagina (vaginitis) | Infiammazione della vagina (vaginite) |
| Inflammation of the vein (phlebitis) | Infiammazione delle vene (flebite) |
| Inflammation of the vulva (vulvitis) | Infiammazione della vulva (vulvite) |
| Inflammation of the windpipe (tracheitis) | Infiammazione della trachea (tracheite) |
| Ingrown nail (onychocryptosis, unguis incarnatus) | Unghia incarnita (onicocriptosi) |
| Inguinal hernia | Ernia inguinale |
| Insecticide poisoning | Avvelenamento da insetticidi |
| Insomnia | Insonnia |
| Intermittent claudication | Claudicatio intermittens |
| Internal bleeding | Emorragia interna |
| Interstitial lung disease | Pneumopatia interstiziale |
| Interstitial nephritis | Nefrite interstiziale |
| Intestinal atresia | Atresia intestinale |
| Intestinal tuberculosis | Tubercolosi intestinale |
| Intracerebral hematoma | Ematoma cerebrale |
| Intracerebral hemorrhage | Emorragia cerebrale |
| Intracranial hypertension | Elevata pressione intracranica |
| Inverted nipple | Capezzolo invertito |
| Involuntary swearing (coprolalia) | Coprolalia |
| Ionising irradiation | Esposizione alle radiazioni ionizzanti |
| Iridodialysis (coredialysis) | Iridodialisi |
| Iritis | Irite |
| Iron deficiency anemia (sideropenic anemia) | Anemia da carenza di ferro |
| Iron poisoning | Avvelenamento da ferro |
| Irritable bowel syndrome (spastic colon) | Sindrome del colon irritabile (colon spastico) |
| Irritant contact dermatitis | Dermatite irritativo da contatto |
| Irritated knee (jumper's knee, patellar tendinopathy) | Peritendite rotulea (ginocchio del saltatore) |
| Ischemia | Ischemia |
| Ischemic heart disease | Ischemia miocardica |
| Ischemic limbs | Ischemia degli arti |
| Ischemic ulceration | Ulcera ischemica |
| Isosporiasis | Isosporiasi |
| Itching | Prurito (pizzicore) |
| Jaundice (icterus) | Ittero (itterizia) |
| Jellyfish sting burn | Ustione da medusa |
| Joint contracture | Contrattura articolare |
| Joint distortion | Distorsione |
| Joint pain (arthralgia) | Articolazione doloroso (artralgia) |
| Joint stiffness | Rigidità dell'articolazione |
| Juvenile osteochondrosis | Osteocondrite dissecante |
| Juvenile rheumatoid arthritis | Artrite idiopatica giovanile |
| Kala-azar (black fever) | Kala-azar (febbre d'Assam, splenomegalia infantile) |
| Kaposi's sarcoma | Sarcoma di Kaposi |
| Kawasaki disease | Sindrome di Kawasaki |
| Keloid | Cheloide |
| Keratosis | Cheratosi |
| Kernicterus | Kernittero (encefalopatia bilirubinica) |
| Kidney failure (renal insufficiency) | Insufficienza renale |
| Kidney stone (nephrolithiasis) | Calcolosi renale (nefrolitiasi) |
| Kidney transplatation | Trapianto renale |
| Kienböck's disease | Morbo di Kienböck |
| Kleptomania | Cleptomania |
| Knee arthrosis | Artrosi di ginocchio |
| Knee dislocation (luxation of the knee) | Lussazione del ginocchio |
| Knock knees (genu valgum) | Ginocchio valgo |

| | |
|---|---|
| Knot (lump) | Nodo (nodulo) |
| Köhler disease | Malattia di Köhler |
| Koplik's spots | Macchie di Koplik |
| Kuru | Kuru |
| Kussmaul breathing | Respiro di Kussmaul |
| Kyphoscoliosis | Cifoscoliosi |
| Kyphosis | Cifosi |
| Laceration (tear) | Lacerazione (strappo) |
| Lack of coordination of muscle movements (ataxia) | Disturbo della coordinazione muscolare (atassia) |
| Lactose intolerance | Intolleranza al lattosio |
| Lambliasis (giardiasis) | Giardiasi (lambliasi) |
| Laryngospasm | Laringospasmo |
| Lassa fever | Febbre di Lassa |
| Lazy eye (amblyopia) | Ambliopia |
| Lead poisoning | Avvelenamento da piombo (saturnismo) |
| Leakage of cerebrospinal fluid through the ear | Perdita di liquido cerebrospinale dall'orechio (otoliquorrea) |
| Leakage of cerebrospinal fluid through the nose | Perdita di liquido cerebrospinale dal naso (rinoliquorrea) |
| Learning disability | Disturbo di apprendimento |
| Leg varicose veins | Varici degli arti inferiori |
| Legg-Calvé-Perthes disease | Malattia di Legg-Perthes-Calvé |
| Leiomyoma | Leiomioma |
| Leiomyosarcoma | Leiomiosarcoma |
| Leishmaniasis | Leishmaniosi |
| Leprosy | Lebbra |
| Leptospirosis | Leptospirosi |
| Leukemia | Leucemia |
| Leukocytosis | Leucocitosi |
| Leukodystrophy | Leucodistrofia |
| Leukoplakia | Leucoplachia |
| Leukorrhea | Leucorea |
| Lichen planus | Lichen planus |
| Ligament rupture (torn ligament) | Rottura del legamento |
| Ligament sprain | Stiramento del legamento |
| Limited joint mobility | Ridotta mobilità articolare |
| Limping | Zoppicamento |
| Lipodystrophy | Lipodistrofia |
| Lipoma | Lipoma |
| Liposarcoma | Liposarcoma |
| Listeriosis | Listeriosi |
| Lithium poisoning | Avvelenamento da litio |
| Little league elbow syndrome (LLE syndrome) | Sindrome del tunnel cubitale |
| Liver abscess | Ascesso epatico |
| Liver cirrhosis | Cirrosi |
| Liver insufficiency | Insufficienza epatica |
| Long-lasting painful erection (priapism) | Erezione persistente dolorosa (priapismo) |
| Lordosis | Lordosi |
| Loss of appetite | Mancanza dell'appetito |
| Loss of half of a field of vision (hemianopsia) | Perdita di metà di campo visivo (emianopsia) |
| Loss of language ability (aphasia) | Perdita di abilità di produzione del linguaggio verbale (afasia) |
| Loss of olfaction (anosmia) | Incapacità di percipire gli odori (disosmia) |
| Loss of strenght (asthenia) | Riduzione della forza muscolare (astenia) |
| Loss of the sense of taste (ageusia) | Incapacità di percipire i sapori (ageusia) |
| Loss of the sense of touch | Perdita di senso di tocco |
| Low back pain (lumbago, lumbo-sacral syndrome) | Lombaggine |
| Low blood pressure (hypotension) | Bassa pressione arteriosa (ipotensione) |
| Low semen volume (oligospermia) | Produzione di pochi spermatozoi (oligospermia) |
| Luetic osteomyelitis | Osteomielite luetica |
| Lung abscess | Ascesso polmonare |
| Lupus erythematosus | Lupus eritematoso sistemico |
| Luxating patella (trick knee, floating patella) | Lussazione della rotula |
| Lyme disease (lyme borreliosis) | Malattia di Lyme (borreliosi di Lyme) |
| Lymphangioma | Linfangioma |
| Lymphangiosarcoma | Linfangiosarcoma |
| Lymphatic leukemia | Leucemia linfatica |
| Lymphedema | Linfedema |
| Lymphocytic choriomeningitis | Coriomeningite linfocitaria |
| Lymphoma | Linfoma |
| Macular degeneration | Degenerazione maculare |
| Madelung's deformity | Deformità di Madelung |
| Malabsorption | Malassorbimento |
| Malaria | Malaria |

| | |
|---|---|
| Malignant hypertension | Ipertensione maligna |
| Malignant mixed tumor | Tumore misto maligno |
| Malignant tumor (cancer) | Tumore maligno |
| Mandibular dislocation | Lussazione della mandibola |
| Mania | Mania |
| Marburg hemorrhagic fever | Febbre emorragica di Marburg |
| Marfan syndrome | Sindrome di Marfan |
| Mastopathy | Mastopatia |
| McCune-Albright syndrome | Sindrome di McCune-Albright-Sternberg |
| Measles | Morbillo |
| Mechanic icterus (bile duct obstruction) | Ittero ostruttivo |
| Mechanical injuries | Lesioni meccaniche |
| Medication overdose | Overdose di farmaci |
| Medullary carcinoma | Carcinoma midollare |
| Medulloblastoma | Medulloblastoma |
| Megacolon | Megacolon |
| Megaloblastic anemia | Anemia megaloblastica |
| Melanoma | Melanoma |
| Melasma (chloasma faciei) | Melasma |
| Melioidosis (Whitmore disease) | Melioidosi |
| Memory loss | Perdita di memoria |
| Meniere's disease | Sindrome di Menière |
| Meningioma | Meningioma |
| Meningocele | Meningocele |
| Meningoencephalocele | Meningoencefalocele |
| Meningomyelocele | Mielomeningocele |
| Meniscal disease | Meniscopatia |
| Meniscus rupture (meniscus tear) | Rottura del menisco |
| Menopause | Menopausa |
| Menstrual disorder | Disturbi mestruali |
| Mental retardation | Ritardo mentale |
| Mercury poisoning | Avvelenamento da mercurio |
| Mesothelioma | Mesotelioma |
| Metabolic acidosis | Acidosi metabolica |
| Metal fume fever | Febbre da inalazione di fumi metallici |
| Metastasis | Metastasi |
| Metatarsalgia (Morton's neuroma) | Metatarsalgia |
| Meteoropathy | Meteoropatia |
| Methanol poisoning | Avvelenamento da metanolo |
| Migraine | Emicrania |
| Milia (milk spots) | Acne miliare |
| Miliaria rubra (sweat rash) | Miliaria rubra |
| Mitral stenosis | Stenosi mitralica |
| Mixed tumor | Tumore misto |
| Molluscum contagiosum | Mollusco contagioso |
| Monocytic leukemia | Leucemia monocitica |
| Mood swing | Cambiamento d'umore |
| Morquio's syndrome (mucopolysaccharidosis IV) | Malattia di Morquio (mucopolisaccaridosi IV) |
| Motor neurone disease | Malattia del motoneurone |
| Movement ability | Abilità di muoversi |
| Movement disorder | Disordine del movimento |
| Movement inability | Mancanza di movimento |
| MRSA | MSSA (MRSA) |
| Mucocele | Mucocele |
| Mucopolysaccharidosis | Mucopolisaccaridosi |
| Mucus in stool | Muco nelle feci |
| Multiple sclerosis | Sclerosi multipla |
| Multiple system atrophy | Atrofia multisistemica |
| Mumps (epidemic parotitis) | Parotite (orecchioni) |
| Murine typhus (endemic typhus) | Tifo murino (tifo endemico) |
| Muscle pain (myalgia) | Dolore muscolare (mialgia) |
| Muscle rupture | Rottura muscolare |
| Muscle strain (muscle pull) | Strappo muscolare |
| Muscle twitch (fasciculation) | Scossa muscolare (fasciciolazione) |
| Muscular contracture | Contrattura muscolare |
| Muscular cramp (spasm) | Spasmo muscolare |
| Muscular dystrophy | Distrofia muscolare |
| Muscular fibrositis | Fibrosite muscolare |
| Muscular hypotonia | Ipotonia muscolare |
| Mushroom poisoning | Avvelenamento da funghi |
| Myasthenia gravis | Miastenia gravis |
| Mycetoma | Micetoma |
| Mycosis | Micosi |
| Myelodysplastic syndrome | Sindrome mielodisplasica |
| Myeloid leukemia | Leucemia mieloide |
| Myoblastoma | Mioblastoma |
| Myoclonic twitches (myoclonus) | Mioclono |
| Myogelosis | Miogelosi |
| Myoma | Mioma |
| Myosarcoma | Miosarcoma |
| Myositis ossificans | Miosite ossificante |

| | |
|---|---|
| Myositis ossificans progressiva | Miosite ossificante progressiva |
| Myxedema | Mixedema |
| Myxoma | Mixoma |
| Myxosarcoma | Mixosarcoma |
| Nail biting (onychophagia) | Abitudine di mangiare le unghie (onicofagia) |
| Narcolepsy | Narcolessia |
| Nasal congestion (stuffy nose) | Congestione nasale |
| Nasal polyp | Polipo nasale |
| Nasal secretion (mucus) | Muco nasale |
| Nasal septum deviation | Deviazione del setto nasale |
| Natural death | Morte naturale |
| Nausea | Nausea |
| Neck myalgia | Mialgia cervicale |
| Neck varicose veins | Vene varicose del collo |
| Necrosis | Necrosi |
| Necrotizing fasciitis | Fascite necrotizzante |
| Neonatal jaundice | Ittero neonatale |
| Nephrosis | Nefrosi |
| Nephrotic syndrome | Sindrome nefrosica |
| Nerve compression (pinched nerve) | Compressone del nervo |
| Nerve lesion | Lesione del nervo |
| Neuralgia | Nevralgia |
| Neurasthenia | Nevrastenia |
| Neurinoma | Neurinoma (Schwannoma) |
| Neuroblastoma | Neuroblastoma |
| Neuroborreliosis | Neuroborreliosi |
| Neurofibromatosis type 1 (Von Recklinghausen's disease) | Neurofibromatosi di tipo1 (malattia di von Recklinghausen) |
| Neurogenic shock | Shock neurogeno |
| Neuroma | Neuroma |
| Neuropathy | Neuropatia |
| Neurosis | Nevrosi |
| Night blindness (nyctalopia) | Cecità notturna (nictalopia) |
| Night sweats | Sudore notturno |
| Nocturnal leg cramps | Crampo notturno alle gambe |
| Nodular goiter | Gozzo multinodulare |
| Non-Hodgkin's lymphoma | Linfoma non Hodgkin |
| Non-ionising irradiation | Irradiazione non ionizzante |
| Nonpassage of urine | Soppressione della secrezione di urina |
| Nose bleeding (epistaxis) | Epistassi (rinorragia) |
| Nuchal rigidity (stiff neck) | Rigidità nucale |
| Numbness in limbs | Parestesie delle estremità |
| Nummular dermatitis | Dermatite nummulare |
| Nystagmus | Nistagmo |
| Obesity | Obesità |
| Oblique fracture | Frattura obliqua |
| Obstructive lesion of the small intestine | Lesione ostruttiva dell'intestino tenue |
| Obstructive shock | Shock ostruttivo |
| Occipital neuralgia (Arnold's neuralgia) | Nevralgia occipitale (nevralgia di Arnold) |
| Occupational disease | Malattia professionale |
| Oligodendroglioma | Oligodendroglioma |
| Oligomenorrhea | Oligomenorrea |
| Onchocerciasis (river blindness) | Oncocercosi (cecità fluviale) |
| Open fracture (compound fracture) | Frattura aperta (frattura esposta) |
| Optic nerve edema | Papilledema (edema del nervo ottico) |
| Orbital cellulitis | Cellulite orbitale |
| Oroya fever (Carrion's disease) | Febbre di Oroya |
| Osgood-Schlatter disease (rugby knee) | Sindrome di Osgood-Schlatter |
| Osteitis fibrosa cystica | Osteitis fibrosa cistica |
| Osteochondroma | Osteocondroma |
| Osteogenesis imperfecta (brittle bone disease) | Osteogenesi imperfetta |
| Osteoma | Osteoma |
| Osteomalacia | Osteomalacia |
| Osteopetrosis (marble bone disease) | Osteopetrosi (malattia delle ossa di marmo) |
| Osteoporosis | Osteoporosi |
| Osteosarcoma | Osteosarcoma |
| Osteosclerosis | Osteosclerosi |
| Ovarian cyst | Cisti ovarica |
| Ovulation pain (mittelschmerz) | Dolore ovulatorio (mittelschmerz) |
| Paget's disease | Morbo di Paget |
| Pain | Dolore |
| Pain syndrome | Sindrome dolorosa |
| Painful menstruation (dysmenorrhea) | Mestruazione dolorosa (dismenorrea) |
| Painful sexual intercourse (dyspareunia) | Dolore durante rapporto sessuale (dispareunia) |
| Painful swallowing (odynophagia) | Deglutizione dolorosa (odinofagia) |
| Painful urination (strangury) | Minzione dolorosa (stranguria) |
| Paleness (pallor) | Pallore |
| Palpitation | Cardiopalmo (palpitazione) |

| | |
|---|---|
| Pancreatic cyst | Cisti pancreatica |
| Pancreatic lipomatosis | Lipomatosi pancreatica |
| Panic attack | Attaco di panico |
| Panner's disease | Malattia di Panner |
| Papillary carcinoma | Carcinoma papillare |
| Papilloma | Papilloma |
| Pappataci fever (phlebotomus fever, sandfly fever) | Febbre da pappataci (febbre da Flebotomi) |
| Paracetamol poisoning | Avvelenamento da paracetamolo |
| Paracoccidioidomycosis (Brazilian blastomycosis) | Paracoccidioidimicosi (blastomicosi sudamericana) |
| Paragonimiasis | Paragonimiasi |
| Paralysis | Paralisi |
| Paralysis of all limbs and torso (quadriplegia, tetraplegia) | Paralisi dei arti superiori e inferiori (quadriplegia) |
| Paralysis of lower extremities (paraplegia) | Paralisi di parte inferiore del corpo (paraplegia) |
| Paralysis of one half of a body (hemiplegia) | Paralisi di una metà del corpo (emiplegia) |
| Paralysis of symmetrical parts of the body (diplegia) | Paralisi di una parte di corpo simmetrica (diplegia) |
| Paranoia | Paranoia |
| Parasitic disease (parasitosis) | Malattia parassitaria (parassitosi) |
| Paratyphoid fever | Febbre paratifoide |
| Paresis | Paresi |
| Parkinson's disease | Morbo di Parkinson |
| Paronychia | Paronichia |
| Partial dislocation (subluxation) | Lussazione incompleta (sublussazione) |
| Passage of large volumes of urine (polyuria) | Aumentata emissione di urina (poliuria) |
| Passing gas (flatulence, farting) | Miscela di gas (flatulenza) |
| Patau syndrome (trisomy 13) | Sindrome di Patau |
| Patent ductus arteriosus (persistent ductus arteriosus) | Dotto arterioso persistente (ductus arteriosus persistente) |
| Pectus excavatum | Torace a imbuto (petto escavato) |
| Pellegrini-Stieda disease | Malattia di Pellegrini-Stieda |
| Pelvic inflammatory disease | Malattia infiammatoria pelvica |
| Pemphigus | Pemfigo |
| Perforated eardrum (tympanorrhexis) | Perforazione del timpano |
| Perforated ulcer | Ulcera perforata |
| Perianal abscess | Ascesso perianale |
| Pericardial carcinosis | Carcinosi pericardiale |
| Pericardial effusion (hydropericard) | Idropericardio |
| Pericardial tamponade (cardiac tamponade) | Tamponamento cardiaco |
| Perinephric abscess | Ascesso perinefrico |
| Periodic breathing (Cheyne-Stokes respiration) | Respiro di Cheyne-Stokes |
| Periodontitis | Parodontite |
| Peripheral nerve lesion | Lesione del nervo periferico |
| Peritoneal carcinosis | Carcinosi peritoneale |
| Pernicious anemia | Anemia perniciosa |
| Personality changes | Cambiamenti di personalità |
| Personality disorder | Disturbo di personalità |
| Pes calcaneus | Piede calcaneo |
| Pes valgus | Piede piatto valgo (pes valgus) |
| Petechia | Petecchia |
| Peyronie's disease (induratio penis plastica) | Induratio penis plastica (malattia di Peyronie) |
| Phantom pain | Dolore fantomatico |
| Phenylketonuria | Fenilchetonuria |
| Pheochromocytoma | Feocromocitoma |
| Phimosis | Fimosi |
| Phlebothrombosis | Flebotrombosi |
| Phlegmon | Flemmone |
| Phobia | Fobia |
| Photophobia (fear of light) | Fotofobia |
| Pig flu (swine influenza, influenzavirus A subtype H1N1) | Influenza suina |
| Pigeon chest (pectus carinatum) | Petto carenato |
| Pilonidal cyst | Cisti pilonidale |
| Pinta | Pinta |
| Plague (pest) | Peste (pestilenza) |
| Plantar fasciitis | Fasciosi plantare |
| Plasmacytoma (multiple myeloma) | Mieloma multiplo |
| Pleural carcinosis | Carcinosi pleurica |
| Pneumoconiosis | Pneumoconiosi |
| Pneumocystis pneumonia (pneumocystosis) | Polmonite da Pneumocisti |
| Pneumothorax | Pneumotorace |
| Poisoning (toxication) | Avvelenamento (intossicazione) |
| Poliomyelitis (polio, infantile paralysis) | Poliomielite (polio, paralisi infantile) |

| | |
|---|---|
| Pollen allergy | Allergia da poline |
| Polycystic kidney disease | Rene policistico |
| Polycythemia | Policitemia |
| Polydactyly | Polidattilia |
| Polymyalgia rheumatica | Polimialgia reumatica |
| Polymyositis | Polimiosite |
| Polyp | Polipo |
| Popliteus syndrome | Tendinite del popliteo |
| Porphyria | Porfiria |
| Portal hypertension | Ipertensione portale |
| Post-necrotic cirrhosis | Cirrosi post-necrotica |
| Post-thrombotic syndrome | Sindrome post trombotica |
| Post-traumatic headache | Cefalea post-traumatica |
| Posterior ankle impingement syndrome | Sindrome da impingement posteriore di caviglia |
| Posttraumatic stress disorder | Disturbo post traumatico da stress |
| Postural back pain | Mal di schiena su base posturale |
| Postural edema | Edema posturale |
| Precocious puberty (premature puberty) | Pubertà precoce (pubertà prematura) |
| Preiser disease | Sindrome di Preiser |
| Premature ejaculation | Eiaculazione precoce |
| Premature sexual development of the opposite sex | Prematuro sviluppo sessuale del sesso opposto |
| Premature sexual development of the same sex | Prematuro sviluppo sessuale dello stesso sesso |
| Premenstrual syndrome (PMS) | Sindrome premestruale |
| Primary amoebic meningoencephalitis | Meningoencefalite amebica primaria |
| Prinzmetal's angina | Angina di Prinzmetal |
| Proctitis | Proctite |
| Productive cough | Tosse produttiva |
| Progressive muscular dystrophy | Distrofia muscolare progressiva |
| Prostate cancer | Cancro della prostata |
| Prostate carcinoma | Carcinoma della prostata |
| Proteinuria (presence of proteins in urine) | Proteinuria |
| Pseudoepithelioma-tous hyperplasia | Iperplasia pseudo-epiteliomatosa |
| Psittacosis (parrot fever) | Psittacosi (psittacornitosi) |
| Psoriasis | Psoriasi |
| Psoriatic arthritis | Artrite psoriasica |
| Psychic changes | Alterazioni dello stato psishico |
| Psychoneurosis | Psiconevrosi (nevrosi) |
| Psychopathy | Psicopatia |
| Psychosis | Psicosi |
| Pulmonary alveolar proteinosis | Proteinosi alveolare polmonare |
| Pulmonary atelectasis | Atelectasia polmonare |
| Pulmonary congestion | Congestione polmonare |
| Pulmonary echinococcosis | Echinococcosi polmonare |
| Pulmonary edema | Edema polmonare |
| Pulmonary embolism | Embolia polmonare |
| Pulmonary heart disease | Cuore polmonare |
| Pulmonary hypertension | Ipertensione arteriosa polmonare |
| Pulmonary hypoplasia | Ipoplasia del tronco polmonare |
| Pulmonary infarction | Infarto polmonare |
| Pulmonary tuberculosis | Tubercolosi polmonare |
| Pulmonary valve stenosis | Stenosi polmonare |
| Pulsing pain | Dolore pulsante |
| Purpura | Porpora |
| Pus | Pus |
| Pus in sputum | Presenza di pus nello sputo |
| Pus in urine (pyuria) | Presenza di pus nelle urine (piuria) |
| Pustule | Pustola |
| Pyelonephritis (kidney infection) | Pielonefrite |
| Pyloric stenosis | Stenosi pilorica |
| Pylorospasm | Pilorospasmo |
| Pyonephrosis | Pionefrosi |
| Pyromania | Piromania |
| Q fever | Febbre Q |
| Quinsy (peritonsillar abscess) | Ascesso peritonsillare |
| Rabies | Rabbia |
| Radial head fracture (radial capitulum fracture) | Frattura del capitello radiale |
| Radiation poisoning | Avvelenamento da radiazione |
| Radioactive irradiation | Irradiazione radioattiva |
| Radioulnar synostosis | Sinostosi radio-ulnare |
| Radius fracture | Frattura del radio |
| Rapid breathing (tachypnea) | Aumento del ritmo respiratorio (tachipnea) |

| | |
|---|---|
| Rash (eruption, eczema) | Sfogo (eruzione cutanea) |
| Rat bite | Morsicatura di ratto |
| Rat-bite fever | Febbre da morso di ratto |
| Raynaud's disease | Sindrome di Raynaud |
| Reactive arthritis (Reiter's syndrome) | Sindrome di Reiter |
| Rectal prolapse | Prolasso del retto |
| Red colored stool | Feci di colore rosso |
| Red urine | Urina di colore rosso |
| Redness of the skin (erythema) | Eritema |
| Refracturing (repeated fracture) | Frattura ripetuta |
| Relapsing fever | Febbre ricorrente |
| Renal agenesis | Agenesia renale |
| Renal cell carcinoma (hypernephroma) | Carcinoma a cellule renali |
| Renal colic | Colica renale |
| Renal cyst | Cisti renale |
| Renal rickets | Rachitismo renale |
| Renal tuberculosis | Tubercolosi dei reni |
| Renal tubular acidosis | Acidosi renale tubulare |
| Renovacsular hypertension | Ipertensione renale |
| Repetitive strain injury (cumulative trauma disorder) | R.S.I (Repetitive Strain Injury) |
| Respiratory alkalosis | Alcalosi respiratoria |
| Respiratory distress syndrome | Sindrome da distress respiratorio |
| Restrictive cardiomyopathy | Cardiomiopatia restrittiva |
| Reticuloendothelial sarcoma | Reticoloendotelioma (reticolosarcoma) |
| Retinal ablation (retinal detachment) | Distacco di retina |
| Retinal artery occlusion | Occlusione arteria retinica |
| Retinal degeneration | Degenerazione della retina |
| Retinitis pigmentosa (retinal pigment epithelium dystrophy) | Retinite pigmentosa |
| Retinopathy of prematurity (retrolental fibroplasia) | Retinopatia del prematuro |
| Retroperitoneal fibrosis (Ormond's disease) | Fibrosi retroperitoneale |
| Retroverted uterus | Retroflessione uterina |
| Reye's syndrome | Sindrome di Reye |
| Rh incompatibility (hemolytic disease of the newborn) | Eritroblastosi fetale (malattia emolitica del neonato) |
| Rhabdomyoma | Rabdomioma |
| Rhabdomyosarcoma | Rabdomiosarcoma |
| Rheumatic fever | Febbre reumatica |
| Rheumatic heart disease | Cardiopatia reumatica |
| Rheumatoid arthritis | Artrite reumatoide |
| Rhinitis | Rinite |
| Rickets (rachitis) | Rachitismo |
| Rickettsiosis | Rickettsiosi |
| Riedel's thyroiditis | Tiroidite di Riedel |
| Rift Valley fever | Febbre della Rift Valley |
| Ringing in ears (tinnitus) | Ronzio auricolare (acufene, tinnito) |
| Rosacea | Rosacea |
| Rotator cuff rupture (rotator cuff tear) | Rottura della cuffia dei rotatori |
| Rotten tooth | Dente guasto |
| Runny nose (rinorrhea) | Naso che cola (rinorrea) |
| Rupture | Rottura |
| Rupture of urinary bladder | Rottura della vescica urinaria |
| Ruptured spleen | Rottura della milza |
| Salicylate poisoning | Avvelenamento da salicilati |
| Salmonellosis | Salmonellosi |
| Sarcoidosis (sarcoid, Besnier-Boeck disease) | Sarcoidosi |
| Sarcoma | Sarcoma |
| Sarcomatoid mesothelioma | Mesotelioma sarcomatoide |
| Sarcopenia | Sarcopenia |
| Scabies (the itch) | Scabbia (rogna) |
| Scar | Cicatrice (sfregio) |
| Scarlet fever | Scarlattina |
| Schistosomiasis (snail fever) | Schistosomiasi |
| Schizophrenia | Schizofrenia |
| Sciatica | Sciatica |
| Scleroderma | Sclerodermia |
| Sclerosing adenosis | Adenosi sclerosante |
| Scoliosis | Scoliosi |
| Scorpion sting | Puntura di scorpione |
| Scotoma | Scotoma |
| Scratch | Graffio (graffiatura) |
| Scrub typhus (Japanese river fever, Tsutsugamushi fever) | Tsutsugamushi (tifo fluviale giapponese) |
| Scurvy | Scorbuto |
| Seasickness | Mal di mare |
| Sebaceous cyst (wen) | Cisti sebacea |

| | |
|---|---|
| Seborrhea | Seborrea |
| Seborrheic keratosis | Cheratosi seborroica |
| Secondary hypertension (inessential hypertension) | Ipertensione arteriosa secondaria |
| Self-harm | Autolesionismo |
| Semicoma | Semi-coma |
| Sensation of fear | Senso della paura |
| Sensitivity to pain (algesia) | Sensibilità al dolore (algesia) |
| Separated shoulder (acromioclavicular dislocation) | Lussazione acromio-clavicolare |
| Sepsis | Sepsi |
| Septic shock | Shock settico |
| Septicemia | Setticemia |
| Sever's disease | Malattia di Sever |
| Severe acute respiratory syndrome (SARS) | SARS (Sindrome Acuta Respiratoria Severa) |
| Sexual addiction | Dipendenza sessuale |
| Sexual differentiation disorder | Disordine della differenziazione sessuale |
| Sexually transmitted disease | Malattia sessualmente trasmissibile |
| Shallow breathing | Respirazione superficiale |
| Sharp pain | Dolore tagliente |
| Shedding of the skin (desquamation) | Perdita dello strato superiore della pelle (desquamazione) |
| Shellfish poisoning | Avvelenamento da molluschi |
| Shigellosis (bacillary dysentery) | Shigellosi |
| Shin splints | Sindrome da stress tibiale mediale |
| Shivering | Brivido |
| Shock | Collaso circolatorio (shock) |
| Shortness of breath (dyspnea) | Fame d'aria (dispnea, respirazione difficoltosa) |
| Shortsightedness (myopia) | Miopia |
| Shoulder arthrosis | Artrosi gleno-omerale |
| Shoulder impingement syndrome (subacromial impingement syndrome) | Sindrome da conflitto subacromiale (impingement sub-acromiale) |
| Shuffling gait | Barcollamento |
| Sickle-cell disease (sickle-cell anemia) | Anemia drepanocitica |
| Siderosis | Siderosi |
| Sight disorder | Disturbo della vista |
| Silicosis | Silicosi |
| Silo-filler's disease | Malattia dei riempitori dei silos |
| Simple bone fracture | Frattura semplice |
| Sinus headache | Sinusite |
| Sister Mary Joseph nodule | Nodulo di Suor Maria Giuseppa |
| Sjögren's syndrome | Sindrome di Sjögren |
| Skin color changes | Cambiamento di colore della pelle |
| Sleep apnea | Sindrome delle apnee nel sonno |
| Sleeping disorder | Disturbo del sonno |
| Sleepwalking (somnambulism) | Sonnambulismo |
| Slow basal metabolism | Basso metabolismo basale |
| Slow breathing rate (bradypnea) | Riduzione della frequenza respiratoria (bradipnea) |
| Slow psychophysiological responses | Lentezza psicofisica |
| Slow pulse rate (bradycardia) | Riduzione della frequenza cardiaca (bradicardia) |
| Small intestine diverticulum | Diverticolo di Meckel |
| Small pupils | Pupille costrette |
| Smallpox | Variola vera (vaiolo) |
| Snake bite | Morsicatura di serpenti |
| Sneezing | Starnuto |
| Sniffing (sniffle) | Tirare su col naso |
| Soft fibroma (fibroma molle, acrochordon) | Mollusco pendulo (fibroma molle) |
| Somnolence | Sonnolenza |
| Sopor | Stupor |
| Sore throat (inflammation of the throat, pharyngitis) | Mal di gola (infiammazione della faringe, faringite) |
| Spanish flu | Influenza spagnola |
| Spasm (cramp) | Spasmo (contrazione involontaria) |
| Spastic arching position (opisthotonus) | Iperestensione della regione posteriore del tronco (opistotono) |
| Speech difficulty (dysphasia) | Disturbo del linguaggio verbale (afasia) |
| Spermatocele | Spermatocele (cisti spermatica) |
| Spider angioma (spider nevus) | Angioma a ragno |
| Spider bite | Morsicatura di ragno |
| Spina bifida | Spina bifida |

| | |
|---|---|
| Spinal deformity | Degenerazione spinale |
| Spinal disc herniation | Ernia del disco |
| Spinal shock | Shock spinale |
| Spiral fracture | Frattura a spirale |
| Splenomegaly | Splenomegalia |
| Split foot (lobster claw foot, ectrodactyly) | Lobster-claw deformità di piede |
| Spondylitis | Spondilite |
| Spondylolisthesis | Spondilolistesi |
| Spondylosis | Spondilosi |
| Spontaneous fractures | Fratture spontanee |
| Sporotrichosis | Sporotricosi |
| Sports injury | Trauma sportivo |
| Sprengel's deformity | Deformità di Sprengel |
| Squamous cell carcinoma (planocellular carcinoma) | Carcinoma a cellule squamose |
| Stab wound | Ferita da punta |
| Staphylococcal food poisoning | Intossicazione alimentare da stafilococco |
| Starvation | Inedia |
| Stenosis of pulmonary artery | Stenosi dell'arteria polmonare |
| Stiffness | Rigidità |
| Stomach cancer (gastric cancer) | Cancro dello stomaco (cancro gastrico) |
| Stomach growling (borborygmus) | Borborigmo |
| Strabismus | Strabismo |
| Strain (sprain, pull) | Stiramento |
| Strangulation | Strangolamento (strozzamento) |
| Streptococcal pharyngitis | Faringite streptococcica |
| Stress fracture | Frattura da stress |
| Stress urinary incontinence | Incontinenza urinaria da sforzo |
| Stroke (cerebrovascular accident) | Colpo apoplettico |
| Stupor | Stupore |
| Stye (chalazion) | Calazio |
| Subarachnoid hemorrhage | Emorragia subaracnoidea |
| Subcutaneous emphysema | Enfisema sottocutaneo |
| Subdural hematoma | Ematoma subdurale |
| Subdural hemorrhage | Emorragia subdurale |
| Sudden infant death syndrome (crib death, cot death) | Sindrome della morte improvvisa del lattante |
| Sudeck's atrophy | Atrofia di Sudeck |
| Sunstroke (heat stroke) | Insolazione (colpo di sole) |
| Supracondylar femoral fracture | Frattura sovracondiloidea del femore |
| Supracondylar humerus fracture | Frattura sovracondiloidea di omero |
| Supramaleolar fracture of tibia and fibula | Frattura del terzo distale di tibia e perone |
| Surgical shock (postoperative shock) | Shock chirurgico |
| Suspension of external breathing (apnea) | Assenza di respirazione (apnea) |
| Sweating | Sudorazione (traspirazione) |
| Swelling | Gonfiore |
| Swimmer's knee | Ginocchio del nuotatore a rana (stiramento cronico del legamento mediale) |
| Syncope | Sincope |
| Syndactyly | Sindattilia |
| Synovial sarcoma | Sarcoma sinoviale |
| Synovioma | Sinovioma |
| Syphilis | Sifilide (lue) |
| Syringomyelia | Siringomielia |
| Tachycardia | Tachicardia |
| Tarsal tunnel syndrome | Sindrome del tunnel tarsale |
| Tendinosis (chronic tendon injury) | Tendinosi |
| Tendinous fibrositis | Fibrosi tendinea |
| Tendon rupture (torn tendon) | Rottura del tendine |
| Tendon strain | Stiramento del tendine |
| Tennis elbow | Gomito del tennista (epicondilite) |
| Tension headache | Cefalea di tipo tensivo |
| Teratocarcinoma | Teratocarcinoma |
| Teratoma | Teratoma |
| Testicular dysgenesis | Disgenesia gonadica |
| Testicular torsion | Torsione del testicolo |
| Tetanus | Tetano |
| Tetany | Tetania |
| Tetralogy of Fallot | Tetralogia di Fallot |
| Thalassemia | Talassemia |
| Thallium poisoning | Avvelenamento da tallio |
| Thermal injuries | Lesioni termiche |
| Thermal wound | Ferita termica |
| Thermonuclear injuries | Ferite provocate da esplosioni termonucleari |

| | |
|---|---|
| Thirst | Sete |
| Thoracic aortic aneurysm | Aneurisma dell'aorta toracica |
| Thoracic outlet syndrome | Sindrome dello stretto toracico superiore |
| Thrombocytopenia | Trombocitopenia |
| Thromboembolism | Tromboembolia |
| Thrombophlebitis | Tromboflebite |
| Thrombosis | Trombosi |
| Thrombotic thrombocytopenic purpura | Porpora trombotica trombocitopenica |
| Thrush (oral candidiasis) | Mughetto (moniliasi orale) |
| Thumb joint arthritis | Rizartrosi (artrosi dell'articolazione alla base del police) |
| Thyroglossal duct cyst | Cisti del dotto tiroglosso |
| Thyroid cyst | Cisti tiroidea |
| Thyrotoxicosis | Tireotossicosi |
| Tibia stress fracture | Frattura da stress della tibia |
| Tibialis posterior syndrome | Periostite tibiale (sindrome del muscolo tibiale posteriore) |
| Tibialis posterior tendinitis | Tendinite del muscolo tibiale posteriore |
| Tic | Tic |
| Tick-borne meningoencephalitis | Encefalite trasmessa da zecche |
| Tight hamstrings syndrome | Sindrome degli ischio-crurali (sindrome dell'hamstring) |
| 'Tight shoes' sensation | Senso delle scarpe troppo strette |
| Tinea capitis (scalp ringworm) | Tigna (tinea capitis) |
| Tinea corporis | Tinea corporis |
| Tinea versicolor (pityriasis versicolor, haole rot) | Pitiriasi versicolor (tinea versicolor) |
| Tingling | Intormentire |
| Tonic-clonic seizure | Crisi tonico-clonica |
| Toothache | Mal di denti |
| Tourette's syndrome | Sindrome di Tourette |
| Toxocariasis | Toxocariasi |
| Toxoplasmosis | Toxoplasmosi |
| Trachoma | Tracoma |
| Transitional cell carcinoma | Carcinoma transizionale |
| Transposition of aorta | Trasposizione dell'aorta |
| Transposition of pulmonary artery | Trasposizione dell'arteria polmonare |
| Transposition of the great vessels | Trasposizione dei grossi vasi |
| Transverse colon | Colon trasverso |
| Transverse fracture | Frattura trasversale |
| Traumatic shock | Shock traumatico |
| Traveller's thrombosis (economy class syndrome) | Sindrome della classe economica |
| Tremor | Tremito (tremore) |
| Trichinosis (trichinellosis) | Trichinosi |
| Trichomonas vaginalis | Trichomonas vaginalis |
| Trichomoniasis | Trichomoniasi |
| Trifascicular block | Blocco trifascicolare |
| Trigeminal neuralgia | Nevralgia del trigemino |
| Trypanosomiasis | Tripanosomiasi |
| Tuberculosis (TBC) | Tubercolosi (tisi) |
| Tuberculous arthritis | Artrite tubercolare |
| Tuberculous lymphadenitis | Linfadenite tubercolare |
| Tuberculous spondylitis (Pott disease) | Spondilite tubercolare (morbo di Pott) |
| Tubular adenoma | Adenoma tubulare |
| Tularemia (rabbit fever) | Tularemia (febbre dei conigli) |
| Tumor (tumour) | Tumore |
| Tungiasis (nigua, pique) | Tungiasi (tunga penetrans) |
| Turner syndrome | Sindrome di Turner |
| Twinging pain | Dolore pungente |
| Typhoid fever (typhoid) | Febbre tifoide (tifo) |
| Ulcer | Ulcera (ulcerazione) |
| Ulcerative colitis | Rettocolite ulcerosa |
| Umbilical hernia | Ernia ombelicale |
| Unclear urine (foggy urine) | Urine torbide |
| Unconsciousness | Incoscienza (stato di incoscienza) |
| Uncontrolled eye movement (opsoclonus) | Movimenti incontrollati degli occhi (opsoclono) |
| Underfedness (malnutrition) | Sottopeso (grave magrezza) |
| Undescended testicle | Mancata discesa del testicolo |
| Unequal size of pupils (anisocoria) | Diseguaglianza del diametro delle pupille (anisocoria) |
| Upper and/or lower jaw fracture (broken upper/lower jaw) | Frattura della mascella e/o della mandibola |
| Upper respiratory tract infection | Infezione del tratto respiratorio superiore |

| | |
|---|---|
| Uremia (autointoxication due to kidney failure) | Uremia (accumulo nel sangue di sostanze azotate a causa dell'insufficienza renale) |
| Ureteral stone (ureterolithiasis) | Calcolo ureterale |
| Urge to vomit | Impulso a vomitare |
| Urinary burning | Bruciore urinario |
| Urinary incontinence | Incontinenza urinaria |
| Urinary retention (ischuria) | Ritenzione urinaria |
| Urination disorder | Disturbo della minzione |
| Urogenital neoplasm | Neoplasie del tratto urogenitale |
| Urogenital tuberculosis | Tubercolosi urogenitale |
| Uterine bleeding (metrorrhagia) | Perdita di sangue al di fuori della mestruazione (metrorragia) |
| Uterine prolapse (fallen womb) | Prolasso uterino |
| Vaginal discharge | Fuoriuscita vaginale |
| Vaginal spasm (vaginismus) | Spasmo di vagina (vaginismo) |
| Van Neck disease | Malattia di Van Neck |
| Varicocele | Varicocele |
| Varicose veins | Varicosi (varici, malattia varicosa) |
| Vasomotor rhinitis | Rinite vasomotoria |
| Venous bleeding | Emorragia venosa |
| Venous thrombosis | Trombosi venosa |
| Venous ulcer (varicose ulcer) | Ulcera varicosa |
| Ventricular fibrillation | Fibrillazione ventricolare |
| Ventricular hypertrophy | Ipertrofia ventricolare |
| Ventricular septal defect | Difetto del setto ventricolare |
| Vibration disease | Malattia da vibrazioni |
| Violent death | Morte violenta |
| Viral conjictivitis | Congiuntivite virale |
| Viral hemorrhagic fever | Febbre emorragica |
| Viral hepatitis | Epatite virale |
| Viral infection | Infezione virale |
| Viral pneumonia | Polmonite virale |
| Vitamin A deficiency | Carenza di vitamina A |
| Vitamin B1 deficiency | Carenza di vitamina B1 |
| Vitamin B2 deficiency | Carenza di vitamina B2 |
| Vitamin B3 deficiency | Carenza di vitamina B3 |
| Vitamin B12 deficiency | Carenza di vitamina B12 |
| Vitamin C deficiency | Carenza de vitamina C |
| Vitamin D deficiency | Carenza de vitamina D |
| Vitamin deficiency | Carenza di vitamine |
| Vitamin K deficiency | Carenza de vitamina K |
| Vitiligo | Vitiligine |
| Vocal chords polyp | Polipo della corda vocale |
| Voice changes | Cambiamento di voce |
| Volkmann's ischemic contracture | Contrattura ischemica di Volkmann |
| Vomiting | Vomito (emetismo) |
| Vomiting of blood (hematemesis) | Emesi emorragica (ematemesi) |
| Vomiting without nausea (cerebral vomiting) | Vomito senza nausea (vomito a getto, vomito cerebrale) |
| Warfare gases poisoning | Avvelenamento da gas tossico |
| Warm sweaty palms | Palmi delle mani caldi e sudati |
| Wart | Verruca |
| Watery eyes | Occhi lacrimosi |
| Watery stool | Consistenza acquosa delle feci |
| Weakness | Debolezza |
| Weight loss (weight reduction) | Dimagrimento |
| West Nile fever | Febbre del Nilo occidentale |
| Wet gangrene | Gangrena umida |
| Whipple's disease | Morbo di Whipple |
| Whitlow (felon) | Patereccio |
| Whooping cough (pertussis) | Pertosse |
| Wilm's tumor (nephroblastoma) | Tumore di Wilms (nefroblastoma) |
| Withdrawal | Crisi d'astinenza |
| Wound (injury, lesion) | Ferita |
| Wrinkle | Ruga |
| Wrist arthrosis | Artrosi di polso |
| Wry neck (torticollis) | Torcicollo |
| Xanthelasma | Xantelasma |
| Xanthoma | Xantoma |
| Yawn | Sbadiglio |
| Yaws (pian) | Framboesia |
| Yellow fever | Febbre gialla |
| Yellow stool | Feci gialle |
| Yolk sac tumor (endodermal sinus tumor) | Tumore del sacco vitellino |
| Zika fever | Febbre Zika |
| Zoonosis | Zoonosi |

| PHARMACY | FARMACIA |
|---|---|
| Activated carbon | Carbone attivo |
| Adrenaline | Adrenalina |
| Aerosol | Aerosol |
| After meal | Dopo il pasto |
| Alcohol | Alcool |
| Almond oil | Olio di mandorla |
| Aminophylline | Aminofillina |
| Ampicillin | Ampicillina |
| Ampoule | Ampolla (fiala) |
| Analgesic (painkiller) | Analgesico |
| Anesthetic | Anestetico |
| Antacid | Antiacido |
| Anti-diabetic drug | Antidiabetico |
| Anti-inflammatory | Antinfiammatorio |
| Anti-obesity medication | Dimagrante (farmaco antiobesità) |
| Antialcoholic drug | Farmaco anti-alcol |
| Antiallergic drug | Farmaco antiallergico |
| Antianemic | Farmaco antianemico |
| Antiarrhythmic agent | Farmaco antiaritmico |
| Antibiotic | Antibiotico |
| Anticoagulant | Anticoagulante |
| Anticonvulsant | Anticonvulsante |
| Antidepressant | Antidepressivo |
| Antidiarrhoeal drug | Antidiarroici |
| Antidote | Antidoto |
| Antiemetic and motion sickness drug | Antiemetico |
| Antihelminthic | Antielmintici |
| Antihemorrhagic (hemostatic) | Emostatico |
| Antihistamine | Antistaminico |
| Antihypertensive drug | Farmaco antiipertensivo |
| Antimalarial drug | Antimalarico |
| Antimycotic | Antimicotico |
| Antioxidant | Antiossidante (sostanza antiossidante) |
| Antiperspirant | Antidiaforetico |
| Antiprotozoal agent | Farmaco antiprotozoico |
| Antipsychotic | Antipsicotico |
| Antipyretic | Antipiretico |
| Antirheumatic drug | Antireumatico |
| Antiseptic | Antisettico |
| Antiserum | Antisiero |
| Antitoxin | Antitossina |
| Antitubercular agent | Farmaco antitubercolare |
| Antiviral drug | Farmaco antivirale |
| Aspirin | Aspirina |
| At noon | A mezzogiorno |
| Atropine | Atropina |
| Bandage | Bendaggio |
| Barbiturate | Barbiturico |
| Blood pressure meter (sphygmomanometer) | Misuratore di pressione (sfigmomanometro) |
| Boric acid | Acido borico |
| Bronchodilator | Broncodilatatore |
| Caffeine | Caffeina |
| Calcium | Calcio |
| Capsule | Capsula |
| Cardiotonic agent | Cardiotonico |
| Castor oil | Olio di ricino |
| Cephalosporin | Cefalosporina |
| Chamomile | Camomilla |
| Chemotherapy | Chemioterapia |
| Chloramphenicol | Cloramfenicolo |
| Chlorine | Cloro |
| Cobalt | Cobalto |
| Codeine | Codeina |
| Compress | Compressa |
| Condom | Preservativo (profilattico, condom) |
| Contact lenses | Lenti a contatto |
| Contact lenses cleaning solution | Soluzione per pulizia lenti a contatto |
| Contraceptive | Contraccettivo |
| Contraceptive foam | Schiuma anticoncezionale |
| Contraceptive pill (oral contraceptive) | Pillola anticoncezionale |
| Contraceptive sponge | Spugna contraccettiva |
| Copper | Rame |
| Corticosteroid | Corticosteroide |
| Cotton-wool | Ovatta |
| Cytostatic | Citostatico |
| Dental floss | Filo interdentale |
| Denture cleaning solution | Soluzione per pulizia dentiera |
| Diaphragm (Dutch cap) | Diaframma |
| Digestive | Digestivo |
| Diuretic | Diuretico |
| Dose | Dose |
| Drops | Gocce |
| Drug allergy | Allergia a medicamento |
| Drug side-effects | Effetti indesiderati da farmaco |
| Ear drops | Gocce per il mal di orecchi |
| Emulsion | Emulsione |
| Enema (clyster) | Clistere |
| Erythromycin | Eritromicina |
| Essential oil | Olio essenziale (olio eterico) |
| Expectorant | Espettorante |
| Eye drops | Collirio |
| Fentanyl | Fentanyl |
| Foam | Schiuma (spuma) |

| | |
|---|---|
| For external application | Per l'applicazione esterna |
| Gauze sponge | Garza |
| Gel | Gel |
| Gentamicin | Gentamicina |
| Glasses | Occhiali |
| Glucose | Glucosio |
| Gram (gramme) | Grammo |
| Hard contact lens | Lente a contatto rigida |
| Heparin | Eparina |
| Herbal tea | Tisana (infuso di erbe) |
| Home pregnancy test | Test di gravidanza ad uso domiciliare |
| Hormone replacement therapy | Terapia ormonale sostitutiva |
| Hot water bottle | Bouillotte (bouilloire) |
| Hypnotic (soporific) | Ipnotico |
| Immunoglobulin | Immunoglobulina |
| Immunosuppressive | Immunosoppressivo |
| In the evening | La sera |
| In the morning | Di mattina |
| Incontinence pads (adult diapers) | Assorbenti per l'incontinenza |
| Inhalation | Inalazione (farmaco per inalazioni) |
| Injection | Iniezione |
| Insect repellent | Insettifugo |
| Insulin | Insulina |
| Interferon | Interferone |
| International System of Units | Sistema internazionale di unità di misura |
| Iodine | Iodio (tintura di iodio) |
| Iron | Ferro |
| Jojoba oil | Olio di jojoba |
| Laxative | Lassativo |
| Lip balm | Burrocacao |
| Liquid powder | Polvere liquido |
| Litre | Litro |
| Lotion | Lozione |
| Lubricant | Lubrificante |
| Magnesium | Magnesio |
| Manganese | Manganese |
| Medical cannabis | Cannabis terapeutica |
| Medication (remedy, drug) | Medicamento (farmaco, rimedio) |
| Methadone | Metadone |
| Microgram | Microgrammo |
| Milligram (milligramme) | Milligrammo |
| Millilitre | Millilitro |
| Mineral | Minerale |
| Mineral oil | Olio minerale |
| Molybdenum | Molibdeno |
| 'Morning -after' pill (postcoital contraception, emergency contraception) | Pillola del "giorno doppo" (contraccezione postcoitale, contraccezione di emergenza) |
| Morphine | Morfina |
| Mosquito repellent | Repellente antizanzare |
| Mouthwash liquid | Collutorio |
| Mucolytic | Mucolitico |
| Muscle relaxant | Miorilassante |
| Nasal drops | Gocce nasali |
| Needle | Ago |
| Nicotine gum | Gomma da masticare antifumo |
| Nicotine patch | Cerotto antifumo |
| Non-steroidal antiinflammatory drug | Farmaco anti-infiammatore non steroide-FANS |
| Nutrient | Sostanza nutriente (sostanza nutritiva) |
| Nystatin | Nistatina |
| Ointment (fat) | Pomata (unguento) |
| Omega-3 fatty acid | Omega-3 acidi grassi |
| On empty stomach (before the meal) | A digiuno |
| Opioid | Oppioide |
| Orally | Oralmente (per via orale, per bocca) |
| Overdose | Sovradosaggio |
| Oxycodone | Ossicodone |
| Paracetamol | Paracetamolo |
| Paraffin | Paraffina |
| Paste | Pasta |
| Pastille (lozenge) | Pasticca (pastiglia) |
| Penicillin | Penicillina |
| Pharmacist | Farmacista |
| Phosphorus | Fosforo |
| Phytotherapy | Fitoterapia |
| Piece | Pezzo (porzione) |
| Plaster (adhesive strip) | Cerotto |
| Poison | Veleno |
| Potassium | Potassio |
| Potion | Pozione |
| Powder | Polverina (polvere) |
| Prescription | Prescrizione (rimedio prescritto) |
| Psychostimulant | Psicostimulanti |
| Purgative | Purgante (purga) |
| Rectal | Rettale |
| Rinsing | Sciacquatra (risciacquatura) |
| Salicylate | Salicilato |
| Saline solution | Soluzione fisiologica |
| Sanitary pads (sanitary napkins) | Assorbenti igienici |
| Scales | Bilancia |
| Sedative | Sedativo (calmante) |
| Serum | Siero |
| Skin cream | Crema |

| | |
|---|---|
| Soap | Sapone |
| Sodium | Sodio |
| Soft contact lens | Lente a contatto morbida |
| Solution | Soluzione |
| Spasmolytic | Spasmolitico |
| Spermicide | Spermicida |
| Spoon | Cucchiaio |
| Spray | Spruzzo (vaporizzato) |
| Sublingual administration | Sublinguale |
| Sugar substitute | Dolcificante artificiale |
| Sulphonamide | Sulfamidici (sulfonamidici) |
| Sulphur | Zolfo |
| Sunscreen (sunblock) | Filtro solare (crema solare ad alta protezione) |
| Suppository | Supposta |
| Syringe | Siringa per iniezioni |
| Syrup | Sciroppo |
| Tablet | Compressa (pasticca, tavoletta) |
| Tampon | Tampone |
| Tetracycline | Tetraciclina |
| Thermometer | Termometro |
| Tincture | Tintura |
| Tonic | Tonico (ricostituente) |
| Tooth paste | Dentifricio |
| Tramadol | Tramadolo |
| Urinary antiseptic | Antisettico urinario |
| Vaccine | Vaccino |
| Vaginal suppository | Candelette |
| Vasodilatator | Vasodilatatore |
| Viagra (sildenafil citrate) | Viagra (citrato di sildenafil) |
| Vial | Bottiglietta (boccetta) |
| Vitamin | Vitamina |
| Vitamin A (retinol) | Vitamina A (retinolo) |
| Vitamin B1 (thiamin) | Vitamina B1 (tiamina) |
| Vitamin B2 (riboflavin) | Vitamina B2 (riboflavina) |
| Vitamin B3 (niacin) | Vitamina B3 (niacina, vitamina PP) |
| Vitamin B4 (adenine) | Vitamina B4 (adenina) |
| Vitamin B5 (pantothenic acid) | Vitamina B5 (acido pantotenico, vitamina W) |
| Vitamin B6 (pyridoxine) | Vitamina B6 (piridossina) |
| Vitamin B7 (inositol) | Vitamina B7 (inositolo) |
| Vitamin B8 (biotin) | Vitamina B8 (biotina) |
| Vitamin B9 (folic acid) | Vitamina B9 (acido folico) |
| Vitamin B10 (factor-R) | Vitamina B10 (vitamina R) |
| Vitamin B11 (factor-S) | Vitamina B11 (vitamina S) |
| Vitamin B12 (cobalamin) | Vitamina B12 (cobalamina) |
| Vitamin C (L-ascorbic acid) | Vitamina C (acido L-ascorbico) |
| Vitamin D2 (ergocalciferol) | Vitamina D2 (ergocalciferolo) |
| Vitamin D3 (cholecalciferol) | Vitamina D3 (colecalciferolo) |
| Vitamin D4 | Vitamina D4 (diidroergocalciferolo) |
| Vitamin D5 (sitocalciferol) | Vitamina D5 (sitocalciferolo) |
| Vitamin E (tocopherol) | Vitamina E (tocoferolo) |
| Vitamin F (linoleic acid) | Vitamina F (acido linoleico) |
| Vitamin J (choline) | Vitamina J (colina) |
| Vitamin K (phylloquinone) | Vitamina K (fillochinone) |
| Vitamin L1 (anthranilic acid) | Vitamina L1 (acido antranilico) |
| Vitamin P (flavonoids) | Vitamina P (flavonoidi) |
| Water-soluble tablets | Compresse solubili |
| Zinc | Zinco |
| Zinc ointment | Zinco pasta |

## MEDICAL FACILITIES, PROCEDURES AND CARE

## ISTITUZIONI, PROCEDURE E CURE DI MEDICINA

| | |
|---|---|
| Administration of drugs | Somministrazione dei farmaci |
| Airway (cannula) | Cannula |
| Alarm | Allarme |
| Ambu bag valve mask | Pallone autoespandibile |
| Ambulance | Autoambulanza |
| Ambulance (clinic) | Ambulanza |
| Amputation | Amputazione |
| Anesthesia | Anestesia |
| Arthrodesis | Artrodesi |
| Artificial respiration | Respirazione artificiale |
| Autopsy | Autopsia |
| Balance training | Esercizi di equilibrio |
| Bath (wash) | Lavare (fare il bagno) |
| Bathroom | Bagno |
| Bed | Letto |
| Bed rest | Riposo a letto |
| Bite | Addentare |
| Blanket | Schiavina |

| | |
|---|---|
| Blood donation | Donazione del sangue |
| Body positioner | Posizionatore |
| Breakfast | Colazione |
| Breast implant | Protese mammaria |
| Breathing exercises | Esercizi di respirazione |
| Bypass | Bypass |
| Calling of the time of death | Proclamazione del tempo della morte |
| Cardiology | Cardiologia |
| Catheter | Catetere |
| Cause of death | Causa di morte |
| Cauterization | Cauterizzazione |
| Chamber-pot | Vaso da notte (pitale) |
| Chemotherapy | Chemioterapia |
| Circumcision | Circoncisione |
| Cleansing | Purificazione |
| Close | Chiudere |
| Contagious | Contagioso (infettivo) |
| Corpse | Cadavere (salma) |
| Cover | Coperta |
| CPR mask | Maschera per rianimazione |
| Crutch | Gruccia (stampella) |
| Cryoextraction | Crioestrazione |
| Cytology | Citologia |
| Debris | Rottami |
| Defecation | Defecazione |
| Defibrillation | Defibrillazione |
| Defibrillator | Defibrillatore |
| Dental crown | Corona |
| Dental extraction | Estrazione del dente |
| Dental filling | Otturazione odontoiatrica |
| Dentist | Dentista |
| Dentures | Protesi dentale |
| Dermatology | Dermatologia |
| Diagnosis | Diagnosi |
| Dialysis | Dialisi |
| Die | Morire |
| Diet | Dieta (regime dietetico) |
| Digestion | Digestione |
| Dining-room | Sala da pranzo (cenàcolo) |
| Dinner (supper) | Cena |
| Doctor (physician) | Dottore/dottoressa (medico) |
| Doctor's office | Ufficio del medico |
| Donor | Donatore/donatrice |
| Door | Porta |
| Drain tube | Tubo di drenaggio |
| Drainage | Drenaggio |
| Dressing | Fasciatura (bendaggio) |
| Drill | Trapano (trivella) |
| Dynamometer | Dinamometro |
| Electrode | Elettrodo |
| Electrode conductive gel | Gel elettro-conduttivo |
| Electrosurgery | Elettrochirurgia |
| Electrotherapy | Elettroterapia |
| Elevator | Ascensore |
| Emergency medical services | Servizio di urgenza ed emergenza medica |
| Endotracheal tube | Tubo endotracheale |
| Escape chair | Sedia portantina |
| Exercise | Esercizio |
| Facelift (rhytidectomy) | Lift facciale (ritidectomia) |
| Feeding tube | Sonda gastrica per nutrizione |
| First aid | Primo soccorso |
| First aid kit | Cassetta di pronto soccorso |
| Gastric lavage (stomach pumping) | Lavanda gastrica |
| General anesthesia | Anestesia generale |
| General practitioner | Medico di medicina generale (medico di famiglia) |
| Germs | Germi |
| Gerontology | Gerontologia |
| Get changed | Cambiarsi |
| Goniometer | Goniometro |
| Gynecology | Ginecologia |
| Head immobilizer | Fermacapo |
| Health insurance | Assicurazione sanitaria |
| Hearing assist device | Apparecchio acustico |
| Heel and elbow protectors | Talloniere e gomitiere antidecubito |
| Heimlich maneuver (abdominal thrusts) | Manovra di Heimlich |
| Hospital | Ospedale (policlinico) |
| Hospital trolley | Carrello |
| Hydrotherapy | Idroterapia |
| Immunology | Immunologia |
| Incontinence pad | Proteggi materasso cerato |
| Infectious disease unit | Reparto di malattie infettive |
| Infusion | Infusione |
| Infusion stand | Piantana portaflebo |
| Injection | Iniezione |
| Intensive care | Terapia intensiva |
| Intensive care unit | Stanza da terapia intensiva |
| Internal medicine | Medicina interna |
| Intubation | Intubazione |
| Kegel exercise | Esercizi di Kegel |
| Laparoscopic surgery | Chirurgia laparoscopica |
| Laryngeal mask airway | Maschera laringea |
| Laryngoscope | Laringoscopio |

| | |
|---|---|
| Laundry | Lavanderia |
| Light | Luce |
| Liposuction | Liposuzione |
| Litter bin | Pattumiera |
| Liver dialysis | Dialisi epatica |
| Lobotomy | Lobotomia |
| Local anesthesia | Anestesia locale |
| Lunch | Pranzo |
| Manometer cuff | Manicotto di sfigmomanometro |
| Manual de fibrillator | Defibrillatore manuale |
| Mattress | Materasso |
| Medical center | Centro di medicina |
| Morgue (mortuary) | Obitorio (mortorio) |
| Nasal cannula | Cannula nasale |
| Neck immobilizer | Collare cervicale |
| Neurology | Neurologia |
| Night table (bedside table) | Comodino |
| Nightgown | Camicia da notte |
| Nurse | Infermiera /infermiere |
| Nursing (care) | Assistenza infermieristica |
| Occupational therapist | Terapista occupazionale |
| Oncology | Oncologia |
| Open | Aprire |
| Operating room | Sala operatoria |
| Operation (surgery) | Operazione (intervento chirurgico) |
| Ophtalmology ward | Reparto di oftalmologia |
| Oropharyngeal airway | Cannula oro-faringea |
| Orthopedics | Ortopedia |
| Otorhinolaryngology | Otorinolaringoiatria |
| Overbed table | Carrello servitore |
| Oxygen mask | Maschera dell'ossigeno |
| Oxygen storage tank | Serbatoio di ossigeno |
| Pacemaker | Cardiostimolatore (stimolatore cardiaco) |
| Palpation | Palpazione |
| Pathology | Patologia |
| Patient | Paziente (ammalato) |
| Patient's room | Camera di malato |
| Pediatrics | Pediatria |
| Percussion | Percussione |
| Percutaneous coronary intervention (coronary angioplasty) | Angioplastica coronarica |
| Pessary | Pessario |
| Physical therapy | Fisioterapia |
| Physiotherapist | Fisioterapista |
| Pillow | Cuscino |
| Plaster cast (immobilization plaster) | Bendaggio gessato |
| Plastic surgery of the abdomen ("tummy tuck", abdominoplasty) | Procedura di chirurgia plastica dell'addome (addominoplastica) |
| Plastic surgery of the breasts (mammoplasty) | Procedura di chirurgia plastica del seno (mastoplastica) |
| Plastic surgery of the eyelid (blepharoplasty) | Procedura di chirurgia plastica della palpebra (blefaroplastica) |
| Plastic surgery of the nose (rhinoplasty) | Procedura di chirurgia plastica del naso (rinoplastica) |
| Postural drainage | Drenaggio posturale |
| Primary health care | Assistenza sanitaria primaria |
| Protect gloves | Guanti protettivi |
| Protection cap | Cuffietta protettiva |
| Protection face mask | Mascherina di protezione |
| Protection gown | Camicia protettiva |
| Protection shoe cover | Sovrascarpe protettive |
| Psychiatry | Psichiatria |
| Psychologist | Psicologo |
| Pulmonary ward | Reparto polmonare |
| Pyjamas (pajamas) | Pigiama |
| Quarantine | Quarantena |
| Radiation | Radiazione |
| Radiology | Radiologia |
| Reanimation | Rianimazione |
| Reception office | Accettazione |
| Recipient of an organ | Ricevente di trapianto |
| Recover (heal) | Sanare (guarire, recuperare) |
| Recovery | Guarigione (ristabilimento) |
| Rehabilitation (rehab) | Riabilitazione |
| Remission | Remissione |
| Renal dialysis | Dialisi renale |
| Respirator | Respiratore |
| Rhinology | Rinologia |
| Rinse | Sciacquare |
| Scalpel | Scalpello |
| Scissors | Forbici |
| Semi-intensive care | Terapia semi-intensiva |
| Sheet | Lenzuolo |
| Shunt | Shunt |
| Slippers | Ciabatte |
| Sonde | Sonda |
| Spit | Sputare |
| Sponge | Spugna |
| Sterile (aseptic) | Sterile |
| Sterilization | Sterilizzazione |

| | |
|---|---|
| Stethoscop | Stetofonendoscopio |
| Storage | Deposito (magazzino) |
| Stretcher | Barella (lettiga) |
| Suction catheter | Tubo d'aspirazione |
| Suction unit (aspirator) | Aspiratore di secreti |
| Surgery | Chirurgia |
| Surgical opening of a direct airway on the neck (tracheostomy) | Incisione chirurgica della trachea (tracheotomia) |
| Surgical opnening of the cranium (craniotomy) | Apertura chirurgica del cranio (craniotomia) |
| Surgical procedure of formation of stoma (colostomy) | Formazione chirurgica di stomia (colostomia) |
| Surgical procedure on a joint (arthrotomy) | Apertura chirurgica di un articolazione (artrotomia) |
| Surgical procedure on the middle ear (stapedectomy) | Intervento chirurgico dell'orecchio medio (stapedectomia) |
| Surgical procedure on the spine (laminectomy) | Asportazione chirurgica della lamina di vertebre (laminectomia) |
| Surgical procedure on the thalamus (thalamotomy) | Intervento chirurgico delle connessioni talamiche (talamotomia) |
| Surgical removal of a breast (mastectomy) | Asportazione chirurgica della mammella (mastectomia) |
| Surgical removal of a hemorrhoid (hemorrhoidectomy) | Asportazione chirurgica delle emorroidi (emorroidectomia) |
| Surgical removal of a lobe of some organ (lobectomy) | Asportazione chirurgica di struttura lobale di un organo (lobectomia) |
| Surgical removal of a testicle (orchidectomy) | Asportazione chirurgica del testicolo (orchiectomia) |
| Surgical removal of adenoids (adenoidectomy) | Asportazione chirurgica delle adenoidi (adenoidectomia) |
| Surgical removal of one or both adrenal glands (adrenalectomy) | Asportazione chirurgica di uno o etrambi surreni (surrenectomia, adrenalectomia) |
| Surgical removal of stones (lithotomy) | Asportazione chirurgica di calcolo (litotomia) |
| Surgical removal of the aneurysm (aneurysmectomy) | Asportazione chirurgica della sacca aneurismatica (aneurismectomia) |
| Surgical removal of the gallbladder (cholecystectomy) | Asportazione chirurgica della colecisti (colecistectomia) |
| Surgical removal of the larynx (laryngectomy) | Asportazione chirurgica della laringe (laringectomia) |
| Surgical removal of the pancreas (pancreatectomy) | Asportazione chirurgica del pancreas (pancreatectomia) |
| Surgical removal of the prostate gland (prostatectomy) | Asportazione chirurgica della prostata (prostatectomia) |
| Surgical removal of the spleen (splenectomy) | Asportazione chirurgica della milza (splenectomia) |
| Surgical removal of the stomach (gastrectomy) | Asportazione chirurgica dello stomaco (gastrectomia) |
| Surgical removal of the thymus (thymectomy) | Asportazione chirurgica del timo (timectomia) |
| Surgical removal of the thyroid gland (thyroidectomy) | Asportazione chirurgica della tiroide (tiroidectomia) |
| Surgical removal of the uterus (hysterectomy) | Asportazione chirurgica dell'utero (isterectomia) |
| Surgical removal of the vermiform appendix (appendectomy) | Asportazione chirurgica dell'appendice (appendicectomia) |
| Surgical removal of tonsils (tonsillectomy) | Asportazione chirurgica delle tonsille (tonsillectomia) |
| Surgical removal of uterine myomas (myomectomy, fibroidectomy) | Asportazione chirurgica di fibromi nell'utero (miomectomia) |
| Surgical sterilization of a man (vasectomy) | Vasectomia |
| Surgical sterilization of a woman (tubal ligation) | Chiusura delle tube |
| Table (desk) | Tavolo (scrivania) |
| Tea | Tè |
| Teeth polishing | Pulitura dei denti |
| Test tube | Provetta |
| Therapy | Terapia |
| Toilet (lavatory) | Vaso sanitario |

| | | | |
|---|---|---|---|
| Traction | Trazione | Barium enema | Indagini radiologiche del colon con clisma opaco a doppio contrasto |
| Transfusion | Trasfusione | | |
| Transplantation | Trapianto | | |
| Transurethral resection of the prostate | Resezione transuretrale della prostata | | |
| | | Barium meal (upper gastrointestinal series) | Radiografia gastroduodenale con pasto baritato |
| Trauma | Trauma | | |
| Trendelenburg position | Posizione di Trendelenburg | | |
| Tweezers | Pinzette | Benzidine stool test | Prova della benzidina |
| Urination (voiding) | Urinazione | | |
| Urological catheter | Catetere vescicale | Biochemical blood tests | Test biochimici di sangue |
| Urology | Urologia | | |
| Using a toilet | Uso del gabinetto | Biomarker | Biomarcatore |
| Vaccination (inoculation) | Vaccinazione (inoculazione) | Biopsy | Biopsia |
| | | Blood culture | Emocoltura |
| Vaccination schedule | Calendario vaccinale | Blood gas test | Analisi dei gas nel sangue (emogas analisi) |
| Vacuum mattress | Materassino a depressione | | |
| | | Blood pressure monitoring | Misurazione della pressione arteriosa |
| Visit | Visita | | |
| Visitor | Ospite (visitatore /visitatrice) | Blood sugar concetration (glucose level) | Concentrazione del glucosio nel plasma |
| Vital signs monitor | Monitor per parametri vitali | | |
| | | Blood urea nitrogen test (BUN) | Azoto ureico nel sangue (BUN) |
| Waiting-room | Sala d'aspetto | | |
| Walker (walking frame) | Deambulatore (tutore per disabili) | Bone densitometry (dual energy X-ray absorpriometry) | Densità minerale ossea |
| Ward | Padiglione (reparto) | | |
| Wardrobe (cupboard, cabinet) | Armadio (credenza) | Bone marrow biopsy | Biopsia del midollo osseo |
| Wash basin | Secchia | Bone scintigraphy | Scintigrafia ossea |
| Water | Acqua | Bone X-ray (bone radiography) | Radiografia ossea |
| Wheelchair | Sedia a rotelle (carrozzella) | | |
| | | Brain ventricle biopsy | Biopsia cerebrale (biopsia dei ventricoli cerebrali) |
| Window | Finestra | | |
| Wound stitching | Suturare la ferita | | |
| | | Breast examination | Esame della mammella |
| **MEDICAL EXAMS** | **ESAMI MEDICI** | | |
| | | Breast ultrasound | Ecografia mammaria |
| Abdominal ultrasound | Ecografia addominale | Bromsulphalein liver function test | Test dela bromosulfaleina di funzionalità epatica |
| Agglutination tests | Test di agglutinazione | | |
| | | Bronchography | Broncografia |
| Alkaline phosphatase | Fosfatasi alcalina totale | Bronchoscopy | Broncoscopia |
| | | CA 125 (cancer antigen 125) | CA 125 (antigene di carcinoma 125) |
| Alpha-fetoprotein test (AFP test) | Test alfa-fetoproteina | | |
| | | CA 19-9 (carbohydrate antigen) | CA 19-9 (antigene carboidratico) |
| Amniocentesis | Amniocentesi | | |
| Angiography | Angiografia | | |
| Anoscopy | Anoscopia | Carcinoembryonic antigen (CEA) | Antigene carcino-embrionario (CEA) |
| Antibiogram | Antibiogramma | | |
| Aortography | Aortografia | Cardiac catheterization (heart cath, angiocardiography) | Cateterismo cardiaco (angiocardiografia) |
| Arteriography | Arteriografia | | |
| Arthroscopy | Artroscopia | | |
| Aspartate transaminase (SGOT) | Aspartato transaminasi (SGOT) | | |
| | | Cardiac ultrasound (echocardiography) | Ecocardiografia |
| Audiometry | Audiometria | | |
| | | Cardiotocography | Cardiotocografia |
| | | Catheter angiography | Angiografia con cateterismo |

| | |
|---|---|
| Central venous pressure (CVP) | Pressione venosa centrale |
| Cephalometry | Cefalometria |
| Cerebral angiography | Angiografia cerebrale |
| Cerebrospinal fluid analysis | Analisi del liquido cerebro-spinale |
| Cerebrospinal fluid culture | Coltura del liquor |
| Cervical conization | Conizzazione |
| Chest X-ray | Radiografia del torace |
| Cholangiography | Colangiografia |
| Colonoscopy | Colonscopia |
| Colposcopy | Colposcopia |
| Complete blood count | Emocromo (analisi del sangue, esame emocromocitometrico) |
| Computed tomography (CT) | Tomografia computerizzata (TC) |
| Contrast medium | Mezzo di contrasto |
| Coronary catheterization (coronarography) | Coronarografia |
| Cystography | Cistografia |
| Cystoscopy | Cistoscopia |
| Defecography | Defecografia |
| Dental X-ray | Radiografia dentale |
| Dermatoscopy (dermoscopy) | Dermatoscopia (dermoscopia) |
| Differential diagnosis | Diagnosi differenziale |
| Digital subtraction angiography | Angiografia digitale a sottrazione |
| Dilated fundus examination | Esame del fundus oculi |
| DNA analysis | Analisi del DNA |
| Doppler echocardiography | Ecocardiografia doppler |
| Drug induced pupillary dilatation | Dilatazione delle pupille provocando con tropicamide |
| Echoencephalography | Ecoencefalografia |
| Electrocardiography (ECG) | Elettrocardiografia |
| Electroencephalography (EEG) | Elettroencefalografia |
| Electromyography (EMG) | Elettromiografia |
| Electroneurography | Elettroneurografia |
| Electroretinography | Elettroretinografia |
| Endometrial biopsy | Biopsia endometriale |
| Endoscopic retrograde cholangiopancreatography (ERCP) | Colangio-pancreatografia endoscopica retrograda |
| Endoscopy | Endoscopia |
| Enteroscopy | Enteroscopia |
| Ergometry test | Ergometria (ECG sotto sforzo) |
| Erythrocyte sedimentation rate | Velocità di eritrosedimentazione |
| Esophageal manometry | Manometria esofagea |
| Esophagogastroduodenoscopy | Esofagogastroduodenoscopia |
| Fine needle aspiration biopsy | Agoaspirato (biopsia mediante ago sottile) |
| Fluoroscopy | Fluoroscopia |
| Functional magnetic resonance imaging (functional MRI) | Risonanza magnetica funzionale |
| Gastric juice chemical examination | Esame chimico di succo gastrico |
| Gastroscopy | Gastroscopia |
| Glasgow coma scale | Punteggio del coma di Glasgow |
| Glucose urine test | Glucosio nelle urine |
| Gonioscopy | Gonioscopia |
| Gynecological examination | Esame ginecologico |
| HbsAg (Hepatitis B surface antigen) | HbsAg (antigene di superficie dell'epatite B) |
| Hematocrit | Ematocrito |
| Hepatobiliary scintigraphy with technetium -99m | Scintigrafia epatobiliare con tecnezio -99m |
| High intensity focused ultrasound | Ultrasuono ad alta intensità focalizzato |
| Hysterescopy | Isteroscopia |
| Hysterosalpingography | Isterosalpingografia |
| Indirect Coombs test | Test di Coombs indiretto |
| Intravenous biligraphy | Biligrafia venosa |
| Intravenous pyelography | Urografia intravenosa (pielografia intravenosa) |
| Iodine -131 thyroid test | Test di captazione tiroidea dello iodio 131 |
| Joint X-ray (arthrography) | Artrografia |
| Karyotype | Cariotipo |
| Kidney biopsy | Biopsia renale |
| Laboratory (lab) | Laboratorio |
| Laboratory tests | Esami di laboratorio |
| Laparoscopy | Laparoscopia |
| Laryngoscopy | Laringoscopia |
| Liver biopsy | Biopsia epatica |
| Liver function tests | Test di funzionalità epatica |
| Liver ultrasound | Ecografia epatica |
| Lumbar myelography | Mielografia lombare |

| | |
|---|---|
| Lumbar puncture | Puntura lombare (rachicentesi) |
| Lung scintigraphy | Scintigrafia polmonare |
| Lymph node biopsy | Biopsia del linfonodo |
| Lymphography (lymphangiography) | Linfangiografia (linfografia) |
| Magnetic resonance imaging (MRI) | Imaging a risonanza magnetica (risonanza magnetica tomografica) |
| Magnetoencephalography (MEG) | Magnetoencefalografia |
| Mammography | Mammografia (mastografia) |
| Mantoux test (PPD test) | Mantoux test |
| Mediastinoscopy | Mediastinoscopia |
| Microbiological culture | Coltura di microrganismi |
| Myelography | Mielografia |
| Ophtalmoscopy | Oftalmoscopia |
| Oral cholecystography | Colecistografia orale |
| Oral glucose tolerance test (OGTT) | Test orale di tolleranca al glucosio (OGTT, curva da carico orale di glucosio) |
| Otoscopy | Otoscopia |
| Pancreas ultrasound | Ecografia pancreatica |
| Papanicolau test (Pap test) | Test di Papanicolaou (Pap test) |
| Partial thromboplastin time (PTT) | Tempo di tromboplastina parziale |
| Patch test | Patch test |
| Patellar reflex | Riflesso patellare |
| Pelvigraphy | Pelvigrafia |
| Pelvimetry | Pelvimetria |
| Perimetry | Perimetria |
| Phenolsulfonphthalein test (PSP test) | Test alla fenolsulfonftaleina |
| Phlebography | Flebografia |
| Plethysmography | Pletismografia |
| Pleural biopsy | Biopsia pleurica |
| Pneumoencephalography | Pneumoencefalografia |
| Polysomnography (sleep study) | Polisonnografia |
| Positron emission tomography | Tomografia ad emissione di positroni |
| Post-void residual urine volume | Volume urinario residuo |
| Pregnancy test | Test di gravidanza |
| Prostate specific antigen | Semenogelasi (antigene prostatico specifico) |
| Prothrombin time | Tempo di protrombina |
| Pulmonary angiography | Angiografia polmonare |
| Pulse monitoring | Misurazione del polso |
| Pyelography | Urografia |
| Radioisotope scanning (nuclear medicine) | Medicina nucleare |
| Rapid strep test | Test rapido dello streptococco |
| Rectal examination | Esplorazione rettale |
| Rectoscopy | Rettoscopia |
| Refractometry | Rifrattometria |
| Renal scintigraphy | Scintigrafia renale |
| Renal ultrasound | Ecografia renale |
| Retrograde pyelography | Pielografia retrograda |
| Rose Waaler test | Rose Waaler test |
| Semen analysis | Spermiogramma |
| Serology blood tests | Esami sierologici |
| Serum albumin | Seroalbumina |
| Serum bilirubin | Test della bilirubina |
| Serum protein electrophoresis | Elettroforesi delle sieroproteine |
| Sialography | Sialografia (scialografia) |
| Sigmoidoscopy | Sigmoidoscopia |
| Skin allergy testing (prick test) | Test cutaneo per le allergie "prick test" |
| Skin biopsy | Biopsia cutanea |
| Skull X-ray (craniography) | Craniografia |
| Speech audiometry | Audiometria di discorso |
| Spinal angiography | Angiografia spinale |
| Spine X-ray (spine radiography) | Radiografia della colonna vertebrale |
| Spirometry (vital capacity test) | Spirometria (pneumometria) |
| Spleen scintigraphy with technetium -99m | Scintigrafia splenica con tecnezio -99m |
| Sputum culture | Coltura di sputo |
| Stereotactic biopsy | Biopsia stereotassica |
| Suboccipital myelography | Mielografia sotto-occipitale |
| Suboccipital puncture | Puntura suboccipitale |
| Thoracoscopy | Toracoscopia |
| Throat swab culture | Coltura di gola |
| Thyroid biopsy | Biopsia della tiroide |
| Thyroid blood tests | Test di ormoni tiroidei nel sangue |
| Thyroid scintigraphy | Scintigrafia tiroidea |
| Thyroid ultrasound | Ecografia della tiroide |
| Tomography | Tomografia |
| Tonometry | Tonometria |

| | |
|---|---|
| Transthoracic percutaneous fine needle aspiration | Agoaspirato polmonare percutaneo transtoracico |
| Tumor marker | Marker tumorale |
| Tympanocentesis | Timpanocentesi |
| Tympanometry | Timpanometria |
| Ultrasound (medical ultrasonography) | Ecografia |
| Ultrasound of the gallbladder and bile ducts | Ecografia colecisti e vie biliari |
| Urea breath test | Test del respiro (urea breath test) |
| Urea clearance test | Urea clearance (clearance dell'urea) |
| Ureteroscopy | Ureteroscopia |
| Urethrography | Uretrografia |
| Urine chemical analysis | Analisi chimiche delle urine |
| Urine culture | Urinocoltura |
| Urine protein test | Proteine nelle urine |
| Urine specific gravity | Esame delle urine peso specifico |
| Urobilinogen in urine | Urobilinogeno nelle urine |
| Vaginal swab culture | Coltura vaginale |
| Ventriculography | Ventricolografia |
| Weber test | Prova di Weber |
| X-ray (radiography) | Radiografia |

## PREGNANCY AND OBSTETRICS — GRAVIDANZA ED OSTETRICIA

| | |
|---|---|
| Abortifacients | Farmaci abortivi |
| Abortion (pregnancy termination) | Interruzione di gravidanza (aborto) |
| Absence of menstrual period (amenorrhea) | Assenza di mestruazioni (amenorrea) |
| Amniocentesis | Amniocentesi |
| Amnioscopy | Amnioscopia |
| Amniotic fluid | Liquido amniotico |
| Amniotic sac | Amnios |
| Artificial insemination | Fecondazione assistita (fecondazione artificiale) |
| Biological parent | Genitore biologico |
| Biophysical profile of the fetus | Profilo biofisico fetale |
| Birth canal | Canale del parto |
| Blastocyst | Blastocisti |
| Bleeding (haemorrhage) | Emorragia |
| Body length of a newborn | Lunghezza di neonato |
| Braxton Hicks contractons | False contrazioni (contrazioni di Braxton Hicks) |
| Breast | Mammella |
| Breast pump | Pompa tiralatte |
| Breathing | Respirazione |
| Breech | Culatta (deretano) |
| Breech position | Posizione podalica del feto |
| Cardiotocography | Cardiotocografia |
| Cervical dilation | Dilatazione della cervice uterina |
| Cesarean section (C-section) | Taglio cesareo |
| Chadwick's sign | Segno del Chadwick (tinta bluastra alla vagina) |
| Childbirth | Parto |
| Choriocarcinoma | Coriocarcinoma |
| Chorion | Corion (corio) |
| Chorion-gonadotrophin | Gonadotropina corionica |
| Chorionic villi | Villi coriali |
| Chorionic villus sampling | Villocentesi |
| Conception | Concezione |
| Contracted pelvis | Pelvi ristretto |
| Cordocentesis | Cordocentesi |
| Curettage | Raschiamento (curetage) |
| Cut | Tagliare (intersecare) |
| Delivery room | Sala parto |
| Diaper | Pannolino |
| Dizygotic twins (biovular twins) | Gemelli fraterni (gemelli dizigoti) |
| Duration of contraction | Durata di contrazioni |
| Duration of pregnancy | Durata della gravidanza |
| Eclampsia | Eclampsia |
| Ectopic pregnancy (extrauterine pregnancy) | Gravidanza ectopica |
| Edema | Edema |
| Egg donation | Ovodonazione |
| Ejaculation | Eiaculazione |
| Embryo | Embrione |
| Endometrial hyperplasia | Iperplasia endometriale |
| EPH gestosis (preeclampsia) | Preeclampsia (gestosi) |
| Episiotomy | Episiotomia |
| Excessive secretion of saliva (hypersalivation) | Produzione di saliva eccessiva (ipersalivazione) |
| Expulsion of placenta | Espulsione della placenta |
| Expulsion of the baby | Espulsione del feto |
| Fallopian tube (oviduct) | Ovidotto (ovidutto) |
| Father | Padre |

| | |
|---|---|
| Fetal anomalies (fetal abnormalities) | Anomalie di sviluppo fetale (anomalie fetali) |
| Fetal hypotrophy | Ipotrofia fetale |
| Fetal pH-metry | pH-metria fetale |
| Fetal weight (birth mass) | Peso di neonato |
| Fetoscopy | Fetoscopia |
| Fetus | Feto |
| Forceps | Forcipe |
| Full term birth | Parto a termine |
| Gestational diabetes | Diabete gestazionale |
| Graafian follicle | Follicolo di Graaf |
| Gynecology | Ginecologia |
| Habitual abortion (recurrent miscarriage) | Aborto abituale |
| Head | Testa |
| Hemolytic disease of the newborn | Eritroblastosi fetale (malattia emolitica del neonato) |
| High blood pressure (hypertension) | Ipertensione arteriosa sistemica |
| Hymen | Imene |
| Hypertrophy of uterus | Ipertrofia dell'utero |
| Implantation | Impianto |
| In vitro fertilisation | Fertilizzazione in vitro |
| Incubator | Incubatrice |
| Infection | Infezione |
| Infertility | Sterilità |
| Inflammation of the fetal membranes (chorioamnionitis) | Infiammazione del sacco amniotico (corioamniosite) |
| Inflammation of the urinary bladder (cystitis) | Infiammazione della vescica urinaria (cistite) |
| Inner membrane of the uterus (endometrium) | Mucosa interna dell'utero (endometrio) |
| Intensity of contractions | Intensità di contrazione |
| Intracytoplasmatic sperm injection | Iniezione intracitoplasmatica dello spermatozoo |
| Labor contraction frequency | Frequenza di contrazioni uterine |
| Labor contractions | Contrazioni del travaglio |
| Lactation | Lattazione |
| Lactiferous duct | Dotto galattoforo |
| Leg varicose veins | Varici degli arti inferiori |
| Lithopedion (stone baby) | Lithopedion |
| Lochia | Lochi |
| Macrosomia (big baby syndrome) | Macrosomia fetale |
| Maternity blues (baby blues) | Sindrome del terzo giorno (baby blues) |
| Maternity hospital | Clinica ostetrica |
| Meconium | Meconio |
| Meconium aspiration syndrome | Sindrome da aspirazione di meconio |
| Meconium ileus | Malattia di Hirschsprung (ostruzione del colon congenita) |
| Meconium peritonitis | Peritonite da meconio |
| Medically assisted procreation | Procreazione assistita |
| Medication that suppresses premature labor (tocolytic) | Farmaco con lo scopo di arrestare le contrazioni uterine (tocolisi) |
| Menopause | Menopausa |
| Menstrual cycle | Ciclo mestruale |
| Menstruation | Mestruazione |
| Microcephaly | Microcefalia |
| Midwife | Ostetrica (levatrice) |
| Mifepristone | Mifepristone |
| Monozygotic twins (identical twins) | Gemelli identici (gemelli monozigoti) |
| Morula | Morula |
| Mother | Madre |
| Multigravida | Pluripara |
| Multiple pregnancy | Gravidanza gemellare |
| Nausea | Nausea |
| Navel (belly button) | Ombelico |
| Neck | Collo |
| Neonatology | Neonatologia |
| Newborn (infant) | Neonato |
| Nipple | Capezzolo |
| Nuchal scan (nuchal translucency) | Translucenza nucale |
| Obstetrician | Ostetrico |
| Obstetrics | Ostetricia |
| Oogenesis | Ovogenesi |
| Ovarian hyperemia | Iperemia dell'ovaio |
| Ovary | Ovaia (ovario) |
| Ovulation | Ovulazione |
| Ovum | Uovo |
| Parent | Genitore |
| Pathological birth | Parto patologico |
| Pelvimetry | Pelvimetria |
| Placenta | Placenta |
| Placenta accreta | Placenta accreta |
| Placenta previa | Placenta previa |
| Placental abruption | Distacco di placenta (abruptio placentae) |
| Placental estrogen | Estrogeno placentare |
| Placental progesterone | Progesterone placentare |
| Plagiocephaly | Plagiocefalia |
| Postmature birth | Parto post-termine |
| Postnatal (postpartum period, puerperium) | Puerperio |

| | |
|---|---|
| **Postnatal depression (postpartum depression)** | Depressione post-partum |
| **Postpartum psychosis** | Psicosi post-partum |
| **Pregnancy** | Gravidanza (gestazione) |
| **Pregnancy risk factors** | Rischio teratogenico |
| **Premature birth** | Parto pretermine |
| **Premature rupture of membranes** | Rottura precoce delle membrane |
| **Preterm newborn** | Neonato pretermine |
| **Primigravida** | Primipara |
| **Progesterone** | Progesterone |
| **Prolactin** | Prolattina |
| **Prolonged birth** | Parto prolungato |
| **Puerperal fever** | Febbre puerperale |
| **Puerperal mastitis** | Mastite puerperale |
| **Puerperal sepsis** | Sepsi puerperale |
| **Push** | Spingere |
| **Pyelonephritis** | Pielonefrite |
| **Quadruplets** | Quattro gemelli |
| **Rupture of membranes** | Rottura delle membrane |
| **Semen (sperm)** | Seme (sperma) |
| **Sperm bank** | Banca del seme |
| **Sperm viability** | Sopravvivenza di spermatozoo |
| **Spermatozoon (sperm cell)** | Spermatozoo |
| **Spontaneous abortion (miscarriage)** | Aborto spontaneo |
| **Stage of birth** | Fase del parto |
| **Stillborn** | Nato morto |
| **Suckling** | Suzione |
| **Surgical removal of the uterus (hysterectomy)** | Asportazione chirurgica dell'utero (isterectomia) |
| **Surrogate mother (womb mother)** | Surrogazione di maternità |
| **TORCH infections** | Complesso TORCH |
| **Transverse fetal position** | Posizione del feto trasversale |
| **Twins** | Gemelli |
| **Ultrasound (medical ultrasonography)** | Ecografia |
| **Umbilical cord** | Funicolo ombelicale |
| **Umbilical cord prolapse** | Prolasso del funicolo ombelicale |
| **Urinary incontinence** | Incontinenza urinaria |
| **Urinary retention (ischuria)** | Ritenzione urinaria |
| **Uterine anomalies** | Anomalie uterine |
| **Vacuum extractor (ventouse)** | Aspiratore a vuoto |
| **Vagina** | Vagina |
| **Vomiting** | Vomito (emetismo) |
| **Water birth** | Parto nell'acqua |
| **Womb (uterus)** | Utero |

DIZIONARIO DI EMERGENZE MEDICHE

Italiano - Inglese

DICTIONARY OF MEDICAL EMERGENCIES

Italian – English

| NUMERI | NUMBERS |
|---|---|
| Zero | Zero |
| Uno | One |
| Due | Two |
| Tre | Three |
| Quattro | Four |
| Cinque | Five |
| Sei | Six |
| Sette | Seven |
| Otto | Eight |
| Nove | Nine |
| Dieci | Ten |
| Undici | Eleven |
| Dodici | Twelve |
| Tredici | Thirteen |
| Quattordici | Fourteen |
| Quindici | Fifteen |
| Sedici | Sixteen |
| Diciassette | Seventeen |
| Diciotto | Eighteen |
| Diciannove | Nineteen |
| Venti | Twenty |
| Ventuno | Twenty-one |
| Ventidue | Twenty-two |
| Trenta | Thirty |
| Quaranta | Forty |
| Cinquanta | Fifty |
| Sessanta | Sixty |
| Settanta | Seventy |
| Ottanta | Eighty |
| Novanta | Ninety |
| Cento | Hundred |
| Centouno | One hundred and one |
| Centoventitre | One hundred and twenty-three |
| Duecento | Two hundred |
| Trecento | Three hundred |
| Quattrocento | Four hundred |
| Cinquecento | Five hundred |
| Seicento | Six hundred |
| Settecento | Seven hundred |
| Ottocento | Eight hundred |
| Novecento | Nine hundred |
| Mille | Thousand |
| Duemila | Two thousand |
| Un milione | Million |
| Un miliardo | Milliard (billion) |

| ORIENTAMENTO NEL TEMPO | ORIENTATION IN TIME |
|---|---|
| Ieri | Yesterday |
| Oggi | Today |
| Domani | Tomorrow |
| Anno | Year |
| Mese | Month |
| Settimana | Week |
| Giorno | Day |
| Ora | Hour |
| Minuto | Minute |
| Sera | Evening |
| Notte | Night |

| ORIENTAMENTO NELLO SPAZIO | ORIENTATION IN SPACE |
|---|---|
| Su | Up (above) |
| In basso | Down (below) |
| Sinistra | Left |
| Destra | Right |
| Davanti | In front |
| Dietro | Behind |
| Dentro | Inside |
| Fuori | Outside |

| GLI ACCIDENTI, CATASTROFI E ANGOSCIA | ACCIDENTS, CATASTROPHES AND DISTRESS |
|---|---|
| Accidente nucleare | Nuclear accident |
| Acqua | Water |
| Affondamento della nave | Sinking of a ship |
| "Aiuto!" | "Help!" |
| Allarme | Alarm |
| Annegamento | Drowning |
| Annegato | Drowned person |
| Arma | Weapon |
| Arma atomica | Atomic weapons |
| Arma bianca | Cold weapon |
| Arma biologica | Biological weapon |
| Arma chimica | Chemical weapon |
| Arma convenzionale | Conventional weapon |
| Arma da fuoco | Firearm |
| Arma di distruzione di massa | Weapon of mass destruction |
| Arma nucleare | Nuclear weapon |
| Arma nucleare strategica | Strategic nuclear weapon |
| Arma nucleare tattica | Tactical nuclear weapon |
| Armi laser | Laser weapon |
| Armi nucleari, biologiche e chimiche (NBC) | ABC weapons |
| Attacco dei pirati | Pirate attack |
| Attacco di squalo | Shark attack |
| Attacco fisico | Physical assault |
| Attaco | Attack |
| Attentato terroristico | Terrorist attack |
| Banchisa (ghiaccio marino, banchiglia) | Sea ice |
| Batterio | Bacteria |
| Boa di salvataggio | Lifebelt (lifebuoy) |
| Bomba | Bomb |
| Bomba al cobalto (bomba gamma, bomba G) | Cobalt bomb |
| Bomba al neutrone (bomba N) | Neutron bomb |

| | |
|---|---|
| Bomba all'idrogeno (bomba H) | Hidrogen bomb (H-bomb) |
| Bomba atomica (bomba A) | Atomic bomb (A-bomb) |
| Bomba sporca | Dirty bomb |
| Bufera di neve (nevicata) | Snow storm |
| Cadutta (cascata) | Fall |
| Campo minato | Mine field |
| Campo per rifugiati | Refugee camp |
| Cane da ricerca e salvataggio | Search and rescue dog |
| Cellula terroristica | Terrorist cell |
| Chiamata di aiuto | Call for help |
| Collisione | Collision |
| Colpo (botta) | Stroke (hit, blow) |
| Colpo di calore | Heat stroke |
| Combattimento | Fight |
| Cordone | Rope |
| Difesa civile | Civil defense |
| Elicottero | Helicopter (chopper) |
| Eliminazione di mine (sminamento) | Mine clearance (demining) |
| Epidemia | Epidemic |
| Eruzione vulcanica | Volcanic eruption |
| Esplosione | Explosion |
| Esplosivo | Explosive |
| Fiume | River |
| Folgorazione (elettrocuzione) | Electric shock |
| Fuoco | Fire |
| Gas tossico | Poison gas |
| Ghiacciaio | Iceberg |
| Ghiaccio | Ice |
| Giubbotto di salvataggio | Lifejacket (life vest) |
| Grotta | Cave |
| Guerra | War |
| Incaglio di nave | Stranding of a ship |
| Incendio (fuoco) | Fire (conflagration) |
| Incidente aereo | Airplane crash |
| Incidente di traffico | Traffic accident |
| Incidente stradale | Car accident |
| Incursione area | Air attack |
| Infortunio domestico | Domestic accident |
| Infortunio sul lavoro | Occupational accident |
| Inondazione | Flood |
| Inquinamento chimico | Chemical pollution |
| Invasione | Invasion |
| Lago | Lake |
| Lava | Lava |
| Macerie (rovine) | Ruins |
| Mare | Sea |
| Mina | Mine |
| Mina navale | Naval mine |
| Mina terrestre | Land mine |
| Montagna | Mountain |
| Nave | Ship |
| Neurotossina | Neurotoxin |
| Neve | Snow |
| Omicidio (uccisione) | Homicide (murder) |
| Onda di marea | Tidal wave |
| Ostaggio | Hostage |
| Pallottola | Bullet |
| Pandemia | Pandemic |
| Paracadute | Parachute |
| Percossa dal fulmine | Thunderclap |
| Pirata | Pirate |
| Plutonio | Plutonium |
| Radiazione | Radiation |
| Rapimento | Kidnapping |
| Rapina | Robbery |
| Relitto | Ship wreck |
| Ricerca | Search |
| Rifugiato | Refugee |
| Rifugio | Shelter |
| Roccia | Rock |
| Rompighiaccio | Icebreaker |
| Salvataggio | Salvage |
| Salvataggio navale | Marine salvage |
| Salvatore | Rescuer |
| Schiavitù (prigionia) | Slavery |
| Scialuppa | Lifeboat |
| Scoria nucleare (scoria radioattiva) | Nuclear waste (radioactive waste) |
| Segnale di allarme | Alarm signal |
| Shrapnel | Shrapnel |
| SOS richiesta | SOS call |
| Squadra di ricerca e salvataggio | Search and rescue team |
| Suicidio | Suicide |
| Tempesta | Storm |
| Tempesta di sabbia | Sandstorm |
| Terra | Land |
| Terremoto | Earthquake |
| Terrorista | Terrorist |
| Test nucleare | Nuclear weapons testing |
| Tifone | Typhoon |
| Traffico di esseri umani | Human trafficking |
| Tromba marina | Waterspout |
| Tsunami | Tsunami |
| Uragano | Hurricane |
| Uranio | Uranium |
| Uranio arricchito | Enriched uranium |
| Valanga | Avalanche |
| Violenza sessuale | Rape (violation) |
| Virus | Virus |
| Vittima | Victim |

## PARTI DEL CORPO UMANO — PARTS OF THE HUMAN BODY

| | |
|---|---|
| Acetilcolina | Acetylcholine |
| Acido desossiribonucleico (DNA) | Deoxyribonucleic acid (DNA) |

| | |
|---|---|
| Acido gastrico | Gastric acid |
| Acido ribonucleico (ARN) | Ribonucleic acid |
| Addome (ventre, pancia) | Belly (abdomen) |
| Adenoipofisi | Adenohypophysis |
| Adrenalina | Adrenalin (adrenaline) |
| Agglutinine | Agglutinin |
| Agglutinogeno | Agglutinogen |
| Albumina | Albumin |
| Aldosterone | Aldosterone |
| Alveolo | Alveolus |
| Amminoacido | Amino acid |
| Ammoniaca | Ammonia |
| Anello cartilagineo | Cartilage ring |
| Ano | Anus |
| Anulare | Ring finger |
| Aorta | Aorta |
| Aorta addominale | Abdominal aorta |
| Aorta toracica | Thoracic aorta |
| Aponeurosi | Aponeurosis |
| Appendice vermiforme | Vermiform appendix (cecal appaendix) |
| Aracnoide | Arachnoid mater |
| Arteria | Artery |
| Arteria coronaria | Coronary artery |
| Arteria polmonare | Pulmonary artery |
| Arteriola | Arteriole |
| Articolazione | Joint |
| Articolazione del gomito | Elbow joint |
| Articolazione dell'anca | Hip joint |
| Articolazione della spalla | Shoulder joint |
| Arto inferiore | Leg |
| Ascella | Armpit (axilla, underarm) |
| Astrocita | Astrocyte |
| Atrio | Cardiac atrium |
| Avambraccio | Forearm |
| Bacino | Innominate bone (pelvis) |
| Barccio | Upper arm |
| Base del cranio | Skull base |
| Bicipite femorale | Biceps femoris muscle |
| Bile | Gall (bile) |
| Bilirubina | Bilirubin |
| Bocca | Mouth |
| Borsa sierosa | Synovial bursa |
| Braccio | Arm |
| Bronchiolo | Bronchiole |
| Bronco | Bronchus |
| Bulbo (midollo allungato, encefalo) | Medulla oblongata |
| Bulbo oculare | Eyeball |
| Calcagno | Calcaneus |
| Calcitonina | Calcitonin |
| Canale di Schlemm | Canal of Schlemm |
| Canale naso-lacrimale | Nasolacrimal duct (tear duct) |
| Canino | Canine tooth |
| Capelli | Hair |
| Capezzolo | Nipple |
| Capillare | Capillary |
| Capsula articolare | Articular capsule (joint capsule) |
| Carboidrato (glucide) | Carbohydrate |
| Carpo | Carpus |
| Cartilagine | Cartilage |
| Cartilagine articolare | Joint cartilage |
| Cassa del timpano | Tympanic cavity |
| Catecolamina | Catecholamine |
| Caviglia | Ankle joint |
| Cavità orale | Mouth cavity (oral cavity) |
| Cellula | Cell |
| Cemento | Cementum |
| Cerume | Earwax (cerumen) |
| Cervelletto | Cerebellum |
| Cervello | Brain |
| Cheratina | Keratin |
| Ciglia | Eyelash |
| Cistifellea | Gall bladder |
| Clavicola | Collarbone (clavicle) |
| Clitoride | Clitoris |
| Coccige | Tailbone (coccyx) |
| Coclea | Cochlea |
| Coledoco | Bile duct |
| Colesterolo | Cholesterol |
| Collagene | Collagen |
| Collo | Neck |
| Colonna vertebrale | Spine (spinal column, backbone) |
| Corda vocale | Vocal chord |
| Cornea | Cornea |
| Coroide | Choroid |
| Corona del dente | Crown of a tooth |
| Corpo luteo | Corpus luteum |
| Corteccia cerebrale | Cerebral cortex |
| Corticosteroide | Corticosteroid |
| Corticosterone | Corticosterone |
| Corticotropina (ormone adrenocorticotropo) | Corticotropin (adrenocorticotropic hormone) |
| Cortisolo | Cortisol |
| Cortisone | Cortisone |
| Coscia | Thigh |
| Costola (costa) | Rib |
| Cotile (acetabolo) | Acetabulum |
| Cranio | Skull |
| Cristallino | Lens |
| Cuoio capelluto | Scalp |
| Cuore | Heart |
| Dendrite | Dendrite |
| Dente | Tooth |
| Dente da latte | Milk tooth |
| Dentina | Dentin |
| Diencefalo | Diencephalon |

| | |
|---|---|
| Digiuno | Jejunum |
| Disco intervertebrale | Intervertebral disc |
| Dito del piede | Toe |
| Dito della mano | Finger |
| Dito indice | Forefinger |
| Dito medio | Middle finger |
| Dotto eiaculatore | Ejaculatory duct |
| Duodeno | Duodenum |
| Dura madre (pachimeninge) | Dura mater |
| Elastina | Elastin |
| Elettrolita | Electrolyte |
| Emoglobina | Hemoglobin |
| Eosinofilo | Eosinophil |
| Epididimo | Epididymis |
| Eritrocita (globulo rosso) | Erythrocyte (red blood cell) |
| Esofago | Gullet (oesophagus) |
| Estradiolo | Estradiol |
| Estrogeno | Estrogen |
| Falange | Phalanx bone |
| Faringe | Pharynx (gullet, gorge) |
| Fascia muscolare | Muscular fascia |
| Fascio di His | Bundle of His |
| Fattore Rh negativo | Rh factor negative |
| Fattore Rh positivo | Rh factor positive |
| Feci | Stool (feces) |
| Fegato | Liver |
| Femore | Thighbone (femur) |
| Fibrina | Fibrin |
| Fibrinogeno | Fibrinogen |
| Fibroblasto | Fibroblast |
| Fluido corporale | Body fluid |
| Fosfolipide | Phospholipid |
| Fronte | Forehead |
| Gabbia toracica | Rib cage |
| Gamba | Lower leg |
| Gas | Gas |
| Gengiva | Gums (gingiva) |
| Ghiandola | Gland |
| Ghiandola bulbouretrale (ghiandola di Cowper) | Bulbourethral gland (Cowper's gland) |
| Ghiandola di Bartolini | Bartholin's gland |
| Ghiandola lacrimale | Lachrymal gland |
| Ghiandola pineale (epifisi) | Pineal body (pineal gland, epiphysis) |
| Ghiandola salivare | Salivary gland |
| Ghiandola sebacea | Sebaceous gland |
| Ghiandola sudoripara | Sweat gland |
| Ginocchio | Knee |
| Glande | Glans |
| Glicogeno | Glycogen |
| Globulina | Globulin |
| Glomerulo | Glomerulus |
| Glucagone | Glucagon |
| Glucocorticoide | Glucocorticoid |
| Glucosio | Glucose |
| Gola | Throat |
| Gomito | Elbow |
| Gonade | Sex gland (gonad) |
| Gonadotropina | Gonadotrophin |
| Granulocita | Granulocyte |
| Granulocita basofilo | Basophil granulocyte |
| Gruppo sanguigno | Blood group |
| Gruppo sanguigno A | Blood group A |
| Gruppo sanguigno AB | Blood group AB |
| Gruppo sanguigno B | Blood group B |
| Gruppo sanguigno 0 | Blood group 0 |
| Guancia | Cheek |
| Ileo | Ileum |
| Imene | Hymen |
| Immunoglobulina | Immunoglobulin |
| Incisivo | Incisor |
| Incudine | Anvil (incus) |
| Inguine | Groin |
| Insulina | Insulin |
| Intestino | Intestine |
| Intestino crasso (colon) | Large intestine (colon) |
| Intestino tenue (piccolo intestino) | Small intestine |
| Ipòfisi (ghiandola pituitaria) | Hypophysis (pituitary gland) |
| Ipotalamo | Hypothalamus |
| Iride | Iris |
| Ischio | Ischium |
| Labbro | Lip |
| Lacrima | Tear |
| Laringe | Larynx |
| Legamento | Ligament |
| Leucocita | Leukocyte |
| Linfa | Lymph |
| Linfocita | Lymphocyte |
| Linfonodo | Lymph gland (lymph node) |
| Lingua | Tongue |
| Lipidi | Fat |
| Liquido cefalorachidiano (liquor, liquido cerebrospinale) | Cerebrospinal fluid |
| Liquido extracellulare | Interstitial fluid |
| Liquido sinoviale (sinovia) | Synovial fluid (synovia) |
| Lombo | Loin |
| Mammella | Breast |
| Mandibola | Lower jaw (mandible) |
| Mano | Hand |
| Martello | Hammer (malleus) |

| | |
|---|---|
| Meato acustico esterno | Auditory canal (ear canal) |
| Melanina | Melanin |
| Melatonina | Melatonin |
| Membrana mucosa | Mucous membrane |
| Membrana sinoviale | Synovial membrane |
| Meninge | Meninx |
| Menisco | Meniscus |
| Mento | Chin |
| Metacarpo | Metacarpus |
| Metatarso | Metatarsus |
| Midollo cerebrale | Brain marrow |
| Midollo osseo | Bone marrow |
| Midollo spinale | Spinal cord |
| Mignolo | Little finger (pinky) |
| Milza | Spleen |
| Mineralcorticoide | Mineralcorticoid |
| Miocardio | Cardiac muscle (myocardium) |
| Molare | Molar |
| Monocita | Monocyte |
| Muco | Mucus |
| Mucosa gastrica | Gastric mucous membrane |
| Muscolo | Muscle |
| Muscolo adduttore | Adductor muscle |
| Muscolo bicipite brachiale | Biceps brachii muscle |
| Muscolo brachiale | Brachialis muscle |
| Muscolo ciliare | Ciliary muscle |
| Muscolo deltoide | Deltoid muscle |
| Muscolo diaframma | Diaphragm |
| Muscolo gluteo | Gluteal muscle |
| Muscolo grande pettorale | Pectoralis major muscle |
| Muscolo intercostale | Intercostal muscle |
| Muscolo massetere | Masseter muscle |
| Musculo obliquo dell'addome | Abdominal oblique muscle |
| Muscolo piccolo pettorale | Pectoralis minor muscle |
| Muscolo quadricipite femorale | Quadriceps femoris muscle |
| Muscolo retto dell'addome | Rectus abdominis muscle |
| Muscolo romboide | Rhomboid muscle |
| Muscolo sartorio | Tailor's muscle (sartorius muscle) |
| Muscolo semimembranoso | Semimembranosus muscle |
| Muscolo semitendinoso | Semitendinosus muscle |
| Muscolo striato | Striated muscle |
| Muscolo trapezio | Trapezius muscle |
| Muscolo tricipite del braccio | Triceps brachii muscle |
| Muscolo tricipite della sura | Triceps surae muscle |
| Narice | Nostril |
| Naso | Nose |
| Nervo | Nerve |
| Nervo cranico | Cranial nerve |
| Nervo ottico | Optic nerve |
| Nervo spinale | Spinal nerve |
| Nervo vestibolococleare (nervo stato-acustico) | Acoustic nerve (vestibulocochlear nerve) |
| Nodo atrioventricolare | Atrioventricular node |
| Noradrenalina | Noradrenaline |
| Nuca | Nape (occiput) |
| Occhio | Eye |
| Ombelico | Navel (belly button) |
| Omero | Upper arm bone (humerus) |
| Orbita oculare | Eye orbit |
| Orecchio | Ear |
| Orecchio medio | Middle ear |
| Organo | Organ |
| Ormone | Hormone |
| Ormone antidiuretico (vasopressina) | Antidiuretic hormone (vasopressin) |
| Ormone luteinizzante | Luteinising hormone |
| Ormone melanotropo | Melanotropin |
| Ossitocina | Oxytocin |
| Osso | Bone |
| Osso carpale | Wrist bone (carpal bone) |
| Osso dell'anca | Hip bone |
| Osso etmoide | Ethmoid bone |
| Osso frontale | Frontal bone |
| Osso iliaco | Ilium |
| Osso ioide | Hyoid bone (lingual bone) |
| Osso lacrimale | Lachrymal bone |
| Osso mascellare | Upper jaw (maxilla) |
| Osso metacarpale | Metacarpal bone |
| Osso metatarsale | Metatarsal bone |
| Osso nasale | Nasal bone |
| Osso occipitale | Occipital bone |
| Osso palatino | Palatine bone |
| Osso parietale | Parietal bone |
| Osso sesamoide | Sesamoid bone |
| Osso sfenoide | Sphenoid bone |
| Osso tarsale | Tarsal bone |
| Osso temporale | Temporal bone |
| Osso zigomatico | Zygoma (cheekbone, malar bone) |
| Ovaia | Ovary |
| Padiglione auricolare | Pinna (auricle) |
| Palato | Palate |
| Palato duro (volta palatina) | Hard palate |
| Palato molle | Soft palate |
| Palmo | Palm |
| Palpebra | Eyelid |

| | |
|---|---|
| Pancreas | Pancreas |
| Papilla gustativa | Taste bud |
| Paratiroide | Parathyroid gland |
| Paratormone (ormone paratiroideo) | Parathyroid hormone |
| Parete addominale | Abdominal wall |
| Pelle (cute) | Skin |
| Pelo | Hair |
| Pene | Penis |
| Pericardio | Pericardium |
| Perineo | Perineum |
| Peritoneo | Peritoneum |
| Perone (fibula) | Fibula (calf bone) |
| Pia madre | Pia mater |
| Pianta del piede | Sole |
| Piede | Foot |
| Plasma | Plasma |
| Pleura (pleure) | Pleura |
| Pleura parietale | Parietal pleura |
| Pleura viscerale | Visceral pleura |
| Pollice | Thumb |
| Polmone | Lung |
| Polmoni | Lungs |
| Polpa dentaria | Dental pulp |
| Polpaccio | Calf |
| Polso | Wrist |
| Pomo d'Adamo | Adam's apple |
| Poro | Pore |
| Premolare | Premolar |
| Prepuzio | Foreskin (prepuce) |
| Progesterone | Progesterone |
| Prostata | Prostate |
| Proteina | Protein |
| Pube (osso pubico) | Pubis (pubic bone) |
| Pupilla | Pupil |
| Radice del dente | Root of a tooth |
| Radio | Radius |
| Rene | Kidney |
| Rètina | Retina |
| Rotula (patella) | Kneecap (patella) |
| Saliva | Saliva (spit, slobber) |
| Sangue | Blood |
| Scapola (omoplata) | Shoulder blade (scapula) |
| Scheletro | Skeleton |
| Scheletro della bocca | Jaw |
| Schiena (dorso) | Back |
| Schiena alto | Upper back |
| Sclera | Sclera |
| Sebo | Sebum |
| Seno | Sinus |
| Sfintere | Sphincter |
| Sigma (colon sigmoideo) | Sigmoid colon |
| Sinapsi (bottone sinaptico) | Synapse |
| Sistema nervoso parasimpatico | Parasympathetic nervous system |
| Sistema nervoso simpatico | Sympathetic nervous system |
| Smalto | Tooth enamel |
| Somatotropina | Growth hormone (somatotrophin) |
| Sopracciglio | Eyebrow |
| Spalla | Shoulder |
| Sperma | Semen |
| Spermatozoo | Sperm (spermatozoon) |
| Staffa (columella) | Stirrup (stapes) |
| Sterno | Breastbone (sternum) |
| Stomaco | Stomach |
| Succo gastrico | Gastric juice |
| Succo intestinale | Intestinal juice |
| Succo pancreatico | Pancreatic juice |
| Sudore | Sweat |
| Surrene | Adrenal gland |
| Talamo | Thalamus |
| Tallone | Heel |
| Tarso | Tarsus |
| Telencefalo (cervello) | Cerebrum (telencephalon) |
| Tempia | Temple |
| Tendine | Tendon (sinew) |
| Tessuto | Tissue |
| Tessuto adiposo | Fat tissue |
| Tessuto muscolare liscio | Smooth muscle |
| Testa | Head |
| Testicolo | Testicle |
| Testosterone | Testosterone |
| Tibia | Shinbone (tibia) |
| Timo | Thymus |
| Timpano (membrana timpanica) | Eardrum (tympanic membrane) |
| Tiroide | Thyroid |
| Tirotropina (ormone tireostimolante) | Thyroid-stimulating hormone (TSH, thyrotropin) |
| Tiroxina | Thyroxine |
| Tonsille | Tonsil |
| Torace | Chest |
| Trachea | Windpipe (trachea) |
| Trigliceride | Triglyceride |
| Triiodotironina | Triiodothyronine |
| Trombocita (piastrina) | Thrombocyte |
| Tronco | Trunk (torso) |
| Tronco encefalico | Brain stem |
| Tuba di Falloppio | Fallopian tube (oviduct) |
| Ulna (cubito) | Ulna |
| Unghia | Nail |
| Uovo | Ovum |
| Urea | Urea |
| Uretere | Ureter |
| Uretra | Urethra |
| Urina | Urine |
| Utero | Womb (uterus) |
| Vagina | Vagina |
| Valvola | Valve (valvula) |

| | |
|---|---|
| Valvola cardiaca | Heart valve (cardiac valve) |
| Valvola mitrale (valvola bicuspide) | Mitral valve (bicuspid valve) |
| Valvola semilunare aortica | Aortic valve |
| Valvola tricuspide | Tricuspid valve |
| Vaso linfatico | Lymph vessel |
| Vaso sanguigno | Blood vessel |
| Vena | Vein |
| Vena cava inferiore | Inferior vena cava |
| Vena cava superiore | Superior vena cava |
| Vena porta | Portal vein |
| Ventricolo | Ventricle |
| Ventricolo cardiaco | Cardiac ventricle |
| Ventricolo cerebrale | Brain ventricle |
| Venula | Venule |
| Vertebra | Vertebra |
| Vertebra coccigea | Coccygeal vertebra |
| Vertebra lombare | Lumbar vertebra |
| Vertebra sacrale | Sacral vertebra |
| Vertebra toracica | Thoracic vertebra |
| Vertice della testa | Vertex (crown of head) |
| Vescica urinaria | Urinary bladder |
| Vescicola seminale | Seminal vesicle |
| Vestibolo | Vestibule |
| Villo intestinale | Intestinal villus |
| Viso | Face |
| Vomere | Vomer |
| Vulva | Vulva |

## I SINTOMI, FERITE E MALATTIE

## SYMPTOMS, INJURIES AND DISEASES

| | |
|---|---|
| Abbassamento della pressione del sangue | Blood pressure fall |
| Abilità di muoversi | Movement ability |
| Abitudine di mangiare le unghie (onicofagia) | Nail biting (onychophagia) |
| Abrasione (escoriazione) | Abrasion |
| Abulia | Aboulia (disorder of diminished motivation) |
| Acariasi | Acariasis |
| Acidosi | Acidosis |
| Acidosi metabolica | Metabolic acidosis |
| Acidosi renale tubulare | Renal tubular acidosis |
| Acloridria | Achlorhydria |
| Acne | Acne |
| Acne miliare | Milia (milk spots) |
| Acne volgare (acne) | Acne vulgaris |
| Acondroplasia | Achondroplasia |
| Acrocianosi | Acrocyanosis |
| Acrofobia (paura dei luoghi e levati) | Acrophobia (fear of heights) |
| Acromegalia | Acromegaly |
| Actinomicosi | Actinomycosis |
| Addome acuto | Acute abdomen |
| Adenocarcinoma | Adenocarcinoma |
| Adenoma | Adenoma |
| Adenoma epatocellulare | Hepatocellular adenoma |
| Adenoma tubulare | Tubular adenoma |
| Adenopatia | Adenopathy |
| Adenosi sclerosante | Sclerosing adenosis |
| Affogamento | Drowning |
| Afta (ulcera all'interno della cavità orale) | Aphtha (mouth ulcer) |
| Agenesia (mancanza di un organo) | Agenesis (absence of an organ) |
| Agenesia renale | Renal agenesis |
| Agranulocitosi | Agranulocytosis |
| Albinismo | Albinism |
| Albuminuria | Albuminuria |
| Alcalosi | Alkalosis |
| Alcalosi respiratoria | Respiratory alkalosis |
| Alcolismo | Alcoholism |
| Algodistrofia | Algodystrophy |
| Allergia | Allergy |
| Allergia a farmaci | Drug allergy |
| Allergia a pello di animali | Fur allergy |
| Allergia a polvere | Dust allergy |
| Allergia alimentare | Food allergy |
| Allergia alle piume | Feather allergy |
| Allergia da poline | Pollen allergy |
| Alluce valgo | Bunion |
| Allucinazione | Hallucination |
| Alopecia | Alopecia |
| Alopecia areata | Alopecia areata |
| Alopecia universale | Alopecia universalis |
| Alterazione della conoscenza | Changes in consciousness |
| Alterazioni dello stato psishico | Psychic changes |
| Ambliopia | Lazy eye (amblyopia) |
| Amebiasi | Amebiasis (amebic dysentery) |
| Amiloidosi | Amyloidosis |
| Ammaccatura (ecchimosi) | Bruise (ecchymosis) |
| Amnesia | Amnesia |
| Amputazione | Amputation |
| Anafilassi | Anaphylactic shock |
| Analgesia | Analgesia (loss of pain sensation) |
| Anchilosi | Ankylosis (joint stiffness) |
| Anchilostomiasi | Ancylostomiasis |

| | |
|---|---|
| Androblastoma | Androblastoma (Sertoli-Leydig cell tumor) |
| Anemia | Anemia |
| Anemia aplastica | Aplastic anemia |
| Anemia da carenza di ferro | Iron deficiency anemia (sideropenic anemia) |
| Anemia da malattia cronica | Anemia of chronic disease |
| Anemia drepanocitica | Sickle-cell disease (sickle-cell anemia) |
| Anemia emolitica | Hemolytic anemia |
| Anemia ipocromica | Hypochromic anemia |
| Anemia megaloblastica | Megaloblastic anemia |
| Anemia perniciosa | Pernicious anemia |
| Anencefalia | Anencephaly |
| Aneurisma | Aneurysm (aneurism) |
| Aneurisma aortica | Aortic aneurysm |
| Aneurisma arteriosa congenita alla base dell'encefalo | Congenital aneurysm of arteries at the base of the brain |
| Aneurisma cerebrale | Cerebral aneurysm |
| Aneurisma cerebrale sferica | Ball-shaped aneurysm of the brain artery |
| Aneurisma dell'aorta addominale | Abdominal aortic aneurysm |
| Aneurisma dell'aorta toracica | Thoracic aortic aneurysm |
| Angina | Angina |
| Angina di Prinzmetal | Prinzmetal's angina |
| Angina pectoris | Angina pectoris |
| Angioedema (edema di Quincke, edema angioneurotico) | Angioedema (angioneurotic edema) |
| Angioma | Angioma |
| Angioma a ragno | Spider angioma (spider nevus) |
| Angiosarcoma | Angiosarcoma |
| Anisakidosi | Anisakiasis |
| Anomalia cerebrovascolare | Cerebrovascular anomaly |
| Anomalia di sviluppo del sistema nervoso | Brain development anomaly |
| Anomalie di sviluppo | Development anomalies |
| Anoressia | Anorexia |
| Anormale perdita di sangue durante il ciclo mestruale (menorragia) | Abnormally heavy menstrual period (menorrhagia) |
| Ansia (ansietà) | Anxiety |
| Antrace | Anthrax |
| Antracosi | Anthracosis |
| Anuria (produzione di urina < 100 ml nelle 24 ore) | Anuria (passage of urine < 100 ml in 24 hours) |
| Aplasia | Aplasia |
| Apoplessia | Apoplexy |
| Appendicite acuta | Acute appendicitis |
| Appetito | Appetite |
| Aritmia | Arrhythmia |
| Aritmia cardiaca | Cardiac arrhythmia |
| Arresto cardiaco | Cardiac arrest (cardiopulmonary arrest) |
| Arteriosclerosi | Arteriosclerosis |
| Arterite temporale (arterite di Horton) | Giant cell arteritis (temporal arteritis) |
| Articolazione doloroso (artralgia) | Joint pain (arthralgia) |
| Artrite idiopatica giovanile | Juvenile rheumatoid arthritis |
| Artrite psoriasica | Psoriatic arthritis |
| Artrite reumatoide | Rheumatoid arthritis |
| Artrite settica | Infectious arthritis (septic arthritis) |
| Artrite tubercolare | Tuberculous arthritis |
| Artrogriposi | Arthrogryposis |
| Artropatia | Arthropathy |
| Artropatia emofilica | Hemophiliac arthropathy |
| Artrosi | Arthrosis (osteoarthritis, degenerative arthritis) |
| Artrosi al piede | Foot arthrosis |
| Artrosi della mano | Hand arthrosis |
| Artrosi di anca | Hip arthrosis |
| Artrosi di caviglia | Ankle arthrosis |
| Artrosi di ginocchio | Knee arthrosis |
| Artrosi gleno-omerale | Shoulder arthrosis |
| Artrosi di gomito | Elbow arthrosis |
| Artrosi di polso | Wrist arthrosis |
| Asbestosi | Asbestosis |
| Ascaridiasi | Ascaridosis |
| Ascesso | Abscess |
| Ascesso anale | Anal abscess |
| Ascesso cerebrale | Brain abscess |
| Ascesso di Brodie | Brodie abscess |
| Ascesso epatico | Liver abscess |
| Ascesso perianale | Perianal abscess |
| Ascesso perinefrico | Perinephric abscess |
| Ascesso peritonsillare | Quinsy (peritonsillar abscess) |
| Ascesso polmonare | Lung abscess |
| Ascite | Ascites |
| Asfissia | Asphyxia |
| Asma | Asthma |
| Aspergilloma (micetoma) | Aspergilloma (mycetoma, fungus ball) |
| Aspergillosi | Aspergillosis |

| | |
|---|---|
| Assenza di mestruazioni (amenorrea) | Absence of menstrual period (amenorrhea) |
| Assenza di respirazione (apnea) | Suspension of external breathing (apnea) |
| Astigmatismo | Astigmatism |
| Astrocitoma | Astrocytoma |
| Atassia ereditaria | Hereditary ataxia |
| Atelectasia polmonare | Pulmonary atelectasis |
| Aterosclerosi | Atherosclerosis |
| Atetosi | Athetosis |
| Atonia muscolare | Atony (atonia) |
| Atresia anale | Anal atresia |
| Atresia biliare | Bile duct atresia |
| Atresia duodenale | Duodenal atresia |
| Atresia esofagea | Esophageal atresia |
| Atresia intestinale | Intestinal atresia |
| Atrofia | Atrophy |
| Atrofia di Sudeck | Sudeck's atrophy |
| Atrofia multi-sistemica | Multiple system atrophy |
| Attaco di panico | Panic attack |
| Aumentata emissione di urina (poliuria) | Passage of large volumes of urine (polyuria) |
| Aumento del ritmo respiratorio (tachipnea) | Rapid breathing (tachypnea) |
| Aumento del senso della sete (polidipsia) | Increased thirst senasation (polydipsia) |
| Aumento della distanza fra due parti del corpo (ipertelorismo) | Increased distance between two organs or parts of the body (hypertelorism) |
| Aumento della pelosità (ipertricosi) | Increased hairiness (hypertrichosis) |
| Aumento della sudorazione (iperidrosi) | Excessive sweating (hyperhidrosis) |
| Aumento di perdita di capelli | Increased hair loss |
| Aumento di volume del fegato (epatomegalia) | Enlarged liver (hepatomegaly) |
| Aumento incontrollato dell'appetito (polifagia) | Excessive hunger (polyphagia) |
| Aumento incontrollato di assunzione di cibo (iperfagia) | Abnormally large intake of food (hyperphagia) |
| Autismo | Autism |
| Autolesionismo | Self-harm |
| Aviofobia (paura di volare) | Aviophobia (fear of flying) |
| Avitaminosi | Avitaminosis |
| Avvelenamento (intossicazione) | Poisoning (toxication) |
| Avvelenamento da alcali | Alkali poisoning |
| Avvelenamento da alcool | Alcohol poisoning |
| Avvelenamento da amianto | Asbestos poisoning |
| Avvelenamento da armi chimiche | Chemical warfare poisoning |
| Avvelenamento da arsenico | Arsenic poisoning |
| Avvelenamento da cadmio | Cadmium poisoning |
| Avvelenamento da cianuro | Cyanide poisoning |
| Avvelenamento da cibo | Food poisoning |
| Avvelenamento da ferro | Iron poisoning |
| Avvelenamento da funghi | Mushroom poisoning |
| Avvelenamento da gas | Gas poisoning |
| Avvelenamento da gas tossico | Warfare gases poisoning |
| Avvelenamento da insetticidi | Insecticide poisoning |
| Avvelenamento da litio | Lithium poisoning |
| Avvelenamento da mercurio | Mercury poisoning |
| Avvelenamento da metanolo | Methanol poisoning |
| Avvelenamento da molluschi | Shellfish poisoning |
| Avvelenamento da monossido di carbonio | Carbon monoxide poisoning |
| Avvelenamento da paracetamolo | Paracetamol poisoning |
| Avvelenamento da pesci | Fish poisoning |
| Avvelenamento da piombo (saturnismo) | Lead poisoning |
| Avvelenamento da radiazione | Radiation poisoning |
| Avvelenamento da salicilati | Salicylate poisoning |
| Avvelenamento da tallio | Thallium poisoning |
| Barcollamento | Shuffling gait |
| Barotrauma | Barotrauma |
| Bartonellosi | Bartonellosis |
| Basalioma (carcinoma basocellulare) | Basal cell carcinoma |
| Basofilia | Basophilia |
| Bassa pressione arteriosa (ipotensione) | Low blood pressure (hypotension) |

| | |
|---|---|
| Bassa temperatura corporea (ipotermia) | Decreased body temperature (hypothermia) |
| Basso metabolismo basale | Slow basal metabolism |
| Batteriemia | Bacteremia |
| Batteriuria | Bacteriuria |
| Bissinosi | Byssinosis (Monday fever) |
| Blastoma | Blastoma |
| Blastomicosi | Blastomycosis |
| Blefarite | Blepharitis |
| Blocco atrioventricolare | Atrioventricular block (AV block) |
| Blocco di branca | Bundle branch block |
| Blocco trifascicolare | Trifascicular block |
| Borborigmo | Stomach growling (borborygmus) |
| Borreliosi | Borreliosis |
| Botulismo | Botulism |
| Brachialgia | Brachial syndrome |
| Brivido | Shivering |
| Bronchiectasia | Bronchiectasis |
| Bronchite cronica | Chronic obstructive pulmonary disease |
| Broncopolmonite | Bronchopneumonia |
| Broncospasmo | Bronchospasm |
| Brucellosi | Brucellosis |
| Bruciore di stomaco (pirosi) | Heartburn |
| Bruciore urinario | Urinary burning |
| Bulimia | Bulimia |
| Cachessia | Cachexia |
| Calazio | Stye (chalazion) |
| Calcificazione | Calcification |
| Calcolo biliare | Gallstone (cholelithiasis) |
| Calcolo ureterale | Ureteral stone (ureterolithiasis) |
| Calcolo urinario (urolitiasi) | Bladder stone (urolithiasis) |
| Calcolosi renale (nefrolitiasi) | Kidney stone (nephrolithiasis) |
| Calicosi | Chalicosis |
| Callo (vescica, bolla) | Blister (corn) |
| Callosità (callo) | Callosity (thickening) |
| Cambiamenti della mucosa | Changes in mucous membrane |
| Cambiamenti della sensazione tattile | Changes in tactile sensation |
| Cambiamenti delle sensazoni olfattive | Changes in olfactory sensation |
| Cambiamenti di nevi | Changes in moles |
| Cambiamenti di personalità | Personality changes |
| Cambiamenti nell'appetito | Appetite changes |
| Cambiamenti nella forma delle ossa | Changes in shape of bones |
| Cambiamenti nelle sensazioni del gusto | Changes in taste sensation |
| Cambiamento d'umore | Mood swing |
| Cambiamento di colore della pelle | Skin color changes |
| Cambiamento di voce | Voice changes |
| Cancrena | Gangrene |
| Cancro della cervice uterina | Cervical cancer |
| Cancro della mammella | Breast cancer |
| Cancro della prostata | Prostate cancer |
| Cancro dello stomaco (cancro gastrico) | Stomach cancer (gastric cancer) |
| Candidosi (candidiasi) | Candidiasis (thrush) |
| Capezzolo invertito | Inverted nipple |
| Capogiro (vertigine) | Dizziness (vertigo) |
| Capsulite adesiva | Frozen shoulder (adhesive capsulitis of shoulder) |
| Carbonchio (pustola) | Carbuncle |
| Carcinoide | Carcinoid |
| Carcinoide bronchiale | Bronchial carcinoid |
| Carcinoma | Carcinoma |
| Carcinoma a cellule renali | Renal cell carcinoma (hypernephroma) |
| Carcinoma a cellule squamose | Squamous cell carcinoma (planocellular carcinoma) |
| Carcinoma anaplastico | Anaplastic carcinoma |
| Carcinoma bronchiale | Bronchial carcinoma |
| Carcinoma della cervice uterina | Cervical carcinoma |
| Carcinoma della prostata | Prostate carcinoma |
| Carcinoma embrionale | Embryonal carcinoma |
| Carcinoma endometriale | Endometrial carcinoma |
| Carcinoma epatocellulare | Hepatocellular carcinoma |
| Carcinoma epiteliale | Epithelial carcinoma |
| Carcinoma gastrico | Gastric carcinoma |
| Carcinoma mammario | Breast carcinoma |
| Carcinoma midollare | Medullary carcinoma |
| Carcinoma papillare | Papillary carcinoma |
| Carcinoma transizionale | Transitional cell carcinoma |

| | |
|---|---|
| Carcinosi (carcinomatosi, cancerosi) | Carcinosis |
| Carcinosi pericardiale | Pericardial carcinosis |
| Carcinosi peritoneale | Peritoneal carcinosis |
| Carcinosi pleurica | Pleural carcinosis |
| Cardiomiopatia | Cardiomyopathy |
| Cardiomiopatia dilatativa | Dilated cardiomyopathy |
| Cardiomiopatia ipertrofica | Hypertrophic cardiomyopathy |
| Cardiomiopatia restrittiva | Restrictive cardiomyopathy |
| Cardiomiopatia tossica | Cardiotoxicity |
| Cardiopalmo (palpitazione) | Palpitation |
| Cardiopatia congenita | Congenital heart disease (congenital cardiopathy) |
| Cardiopatia reumatica | Rheumatic heart disease |
| Carenza di estrogeno | Estrogen deficiency |
| Carenza di fattore di coagulazione | Coagulation factor deficiency |
| Carenza di vitamine | Vitamin deficiency |
| Carenza di vitamina A | Vitamin A deficiency |
| Carenza di vitamina B1 | Vitamin B1 deficiency |
| Carenza di vitamina B2 | Vitamin B2 deficiency |
| Carenza di vitamina B3 | Vitamin B3 deficiency |
| Carenza di vitamina B12 | Vitamin B12 deficiency |
| Carenza di vitamina C | Vitamin C deficiency |
| Carenza di vitamina D | Vitamin D deficiency |
| Carenza di vitamina K | Vitamin K deficiency |
| Carie dentaria | Dental caries |
| Catalessia | Catalepsy |
| Cataplessia | Cataplexy |
| Cataratta | Cataract |
| Catarro | Catarrh |
| Cecità | Blindness |
| Cecità notturna (nictalopia) | Night blindness (nyctalopia) |
| Cefalea a grappolo | Cluster headache |
| Cefalea di tipo tensivo | Tension headache |
| Cefalea post-traumatica | Post-traumatic headache |
| Cefalocèle | Cephalocele |
| Celiachia (malattia caliacha) | Coeliac disease (celiac disease) |
| Cellulite | Cellulitis |
| Cellulite orbitale | Orbital cellulitis |
| Cercaria | Cercaria |
| Cheloide | Keloid |
| Cheratosi | Keratosis |
| Cheratosi seborroica | Seborrheic keratosis |
| Cheratosi solare | Actinic keratosis |
| Chetoacidosi diabetica | Diabetic ketoacidosis |
| Chikungunya | Chikungunya |
| Chilotorace | Chylothorax |
| Cianosi | Cyanosis |
| Cicatrice (sfregio) | Scar |
| Cifoscoliosi | Kyphoscoliosis |
| Cifosi | Kyphosis |
| Cirrosi | Liver cirrhosis |
| Cirrosi alcolica | Alcoholic cirrhosis |
| Cirrosi biliare | Biliary cirrhosis |
| Cirrosi criptogenica | Cryptogenic cirrhosis |
| Cirrosi post-necrotica | Post-necrotic cirrhosis |
| Cistadenocarcinoma | Cystadenocarcinoma |
| Cistadenofibroma | Cystadenofibroma |
| Cistadenoma | Cystadenoma |
| Cisti (ciste) | Cyst |
| Cisti del dotto tiroglosso | Thyroglossal duct cyst |
| Cisti dermoide | Dermoid cyst |
| Cisti ovarica | Ovarian cyst |
| Cisti pancreatica | Pancreatic cyst |
| Cisti pilonidale | Pilonidal cyst |
| Cisti renale | Renal cyst |
| Cisti sebacea | Sebaceous cyst (wen) |
| Cisti tiroidea | Thyroid cyst |
| Cisticercosi | Cysticercosis |
| Cistoma | Cystoma |
| Claudicatio intermittens | Intermittent claudication |
| Claustrofobia (paura di luoghi chiusi) | Claustrophobia (fear of closed space) |
| Cleptomania | Kleptomania |
| Clonorchiasi | Clonorchiasis |
| Coagulazione intravascolare disseminata | Disseminated intra-vascular coagulation |
| Coartazione dell'aorta | Coarctation of the aorta |
| Coccidiomicosi | Coccidioidomycosis (San Joaquin Valley fever) |
| Coccigodinia | Coccygodynia |
| Colangiocarcinoma (carcinoma colangiocellulare) | Cholangiocellular carcinoma |
| Colera | Cholera |
| Colica | Colic |
| Colica addominale | Abdominal colic |
| Colica biliare | Biliary colic |

| | |
|---|---|
| Colica renale | Renal colic |
| Coliche del neonato | Baby colic |
| Collaso circolatorio (shock) | Shock |
| Collasso | Collapse |
| Colon trasverso | Transverse colon |
| Colpo apoplettico | Stroke (cerebrovascular accident) |
| Coma | Coma |
| Coma diabetico | Diabetic coma |
| Commozione cerebrale | Brain concussion |
| Compressione cerebrale | Brain compression |
| Compressone del nervo | Nerve compression (pinched nerve) |
| Condiloma | Genital wart |
| Condroblastoma | Chondroblastoma |
| Condroma | Chondroma |
| Condrosarcoma | Chondrosarcoma |
| Confusione (disordine) | Confusion |
| Congelamento | Frostbite |
| Congestione nasale | Nasal congestion (stuffy nose) |
| Congestione polmonare | Pulmonary congestion |
| Congiuntivite allergica | Allergic conjunctivitis |
| Congiuntivite batterica | Bacterial conjunctivitis |
| Congiuntivite irritativa da agenti chimici | Chemical conjunctivitis |
| Congiuntivite irritativa da corpi estranei | Conjunctival foreign body |
| Congiuntivite virale | Viral conjuctivitis |
| Consistenza acquosa delle feci | Watery stool |
| Contrattura | Contracture |
| Contrattura articolare | Joint contracture |
| Contrattura ischemica di Volkmann | Volkmann's ischemic contracture |
| Contrattura muscolare | Muscular contracture |
| Contusione | Contusion |
| Contusione cerebrale | Cerebral contusion |
| Convulsioni | Convulsions |
| Convulsioni febbrili | Febrile convulsions |
| Coprolalìa | Involuntary swearing (coprolalia) |
| Coreoatetosi | Choreoathetosis |
| Coriocarcinoma | Choriocarcinoma |
| Coriomeningite linfocitaria | Lymphocytic choriomeningitis |
| Coronaropatia | Coronary disease |
| Corpo estraneo nel naso | Foreign body in nose |
| Corpo estraneo nell'orecchio | Foreign body in ear |
| Costa cervicale | Cervical rib |
| Crampo notturno alle gambe | Nocturnal leg cramps |
| Crepitazione | Crepitation |
| Criptococcosi | Cryptococcosis |
| Criptorchidismo | Cryptorchidism |
| Crisi d'astinenza | Withdrawal |
| Crisi tonico-clonica | Tonic-clonic seizure |
| Cromomicosi (cromoblastomicosi) | Chromoblastomycosis (chromomycosis, Pedroso's disease) |
| Crosta (escara) | Crust (scab) |
| Croup (laringite acuta ostruttiva) | Croup (acute obstructive laryngitis) |
| Cuore dell'atleta (ipertrofia cardiaca da sport) | Athlete's heart (cardiac hypertrophy) |
| Cuore polmonare | Pulmonary heart disease |
| Cuore polmonare acuto | Acute pulmonary heart |
| Cupololitiasi (canalolitiasi) | Benign positional vertigo |
| Daltonismo | Daltonism |
| Debolezza | Weakness |
| Decompensazione cardiaca | Cardiac decompensation |
| Deformità di Madelung | Madelung's deformity |
| Deformità di Sprengel | Sprengel's deformity |
| Degenerazione della retina | Retinal degeneration |
| Degenerazione maculare | Macular degeneration |
| Degenerazione spinale | Spinal deformity |
| Deglutizione dolorosa (odinofagia) | Painful swallowing (odynophagia) |
| Delirio | Delirium |
| Demenza | Dementia |
| Demineralizzazione | Demineralization |
| Dengue | Dengue fever |
| Dente guasto | Rotten tooth |
| Depressione | Depression |
| Dermatite allergica | Allergic contact dermatitis |
| Dermatite da contatto | Contact dermatitis |
| Dermatite erpetiforme di Duhring | Dermatitis herpetiformis (Duhring's disease) |
| Dermatite irritativo da contatto | Irritant contact dermatitis |
| Dermatite nummulare | Nummular dermatitis |

| | |
|---|---|
| Dermatite seborroica infantile | Cradle cap (infantile seborrhoeic dermatitis) |
| Dermatomicosi | Dermatomycosis |
| Dermatomiosite | Dermatomyositis |
| Deviazione del setto nasale | Nasal septum deviation |
| Diabete | Diabetes |
| Diabete insipido | Diabetes insipidus |
| Diabete mellito | Diabetes mellitus |
| Diabete mellito di tipo 1 | Diabetes mellitus type 1 |
| Diabete mellito di tipo 2 | Diabetes mellitus type 2 |
| Diarrea | Diarrhea |
| Difetto cardiaco congenito | Congenital heart defect |
| Difetto del piede | Foot deformity |
| Difetto del setto interatriale | Atrial septal defect |
| Difetto del setto ventricolare | Ventricular septal defect |
| Difficoltà a defecare (tenesmo) | Difficult defecation (tenesmus) |
| Difficoltà a deglutire (disfagia) | Difficult swallowing (dysphagia) |
| Difterite | Diphtheria |
| Dilatazione gastrica acuta | Acute gastric dilatation |
| Dimagramento | Weight loss (weight reduction) |
| Diminuita escrezione urinaria (oliguria) | Decreased production of urine (oliguria) |
| Dipendenza | Addiction |
| Dipendenza sessuale | Sexual addiction |
| Discartrosi (discopatia degenerativa) | Discarthrosis (degenerative disc disease) |
| Discondroplasia | Dyschondroplasia |
| Diseguaglianza del diametro delle pupille (anisocoria) | Unequal size of pupils (anisocoria) |
| Disgenesia gonadica | Testicular dysgenesis |
| Disgerminoma | Dysgerminoma |
| Disidratazione | Dehydration |
| Disidrosi | Dyshidrosis |
| Dislessia | Dyslexia |
| Dislocazione dei frammenti | Dislocated fragments |
| Disordine della differenziazione sessuale | Sexual differentiation disorder |
| Disordine del movimento | Movement disorder |
| Disorientamento | Disorientation |
| Dispepsia | Dyspepsia (upset stomach) |
| Displasia cervicale | Cervical dysplasia |
| Displasia fibrosa | Fibrous dysplasia |
| Displasia ventricolare destra aritmogena | Arrhytmogenic right ventricular dysplasia |
| Dispnea parossistica notturna | Cardiac asthma (paroxysmal nocturnal dyspnea) |
| Dissecazione aortica | Aortic dissection |
| Dissenteria | Dysentery (flux) |
| Distacco di retina | Retinal ablation (retinal detachment) |
| Distonia | Dystonia |
| Distorsione | Joint distortion |
| Distorsione alla caviglia | Ankle distortion |
| Distrofia | Dystrophy |
| Distrofia di Duchenne | Duchenne muscular dystrophy |
| Distrofia muscolare | Muscular dystrophy |
| Distrofia muscolare progressiva | Progressive muscular dystrophy |
| Disturbi mestruali | Menstrual disorder |
| Disturbo borderline di personalità | Borderline personality disorder |
| Disturbo del comportamento alimentare | Eating disorder |
| Disturbo del linguaggio verbale (afasia) | Speech difficulty (dysphasia) |
| Disturbo del sonno | Sleeping disorder |
| Disturbo dell'equilibrio | Balance disorder |
| Disturbo dell'udito | Hearing disorder |
| Disturbo dell'umore | Behavioral disorder |
| Disturbo della concentrazione | Attention deficit disorder |
| Disturbo della coordinazione muscolare (atassia) | Lack of coordination of muscle movements (ataxia) |
| Disturbo della minzione | Urination disorder |
| Disturbo della vista | Sight disorder |
| Disturbo di apprendimento | Learning disability |
| Disturbo di personalità | Personality disorder |
| Disturbo post traumatico da stress | Posttraumatic stress disorder |
| Dita ippocratiche (dita a bacchetta di tamburo) | Finger clubbing (digital clubbing) |
| Diverticolite | Diverticulitis |
| Diverticolo | Diverticulum |
| Diverticolo del colon | Colon diverticulum |
| Diverticolo di Meckel | Small intestine diverticulum |
| Diverticolo duodenale | Duodenal diverticulum |
| Diverticolosi | Diverticulosis |
| Dolore | Pain |
| Dolore acuto | Acute pain |

| | |
|---|---|
| Dolore addominale | Abdominal pain |
| Dolore al seno (mastalgia) | Breast pain (mastalgia) |
| Dolore auricolare (otalgia) | Ear pain (otalgia) |
| Dolore cronico | Chronic pain |
| Dolore durante rapporto sessuale (dispareunia) | Painful sexual intercourse (dyspareunia) |
| Dolore fantomatico | Phantom pain |
| Dolore muscolare (mialgia) | Muscle pain (myalgia) |
| Dolore ottuso | Dull pain |
| Dolore ovulatorio (mittelschmerz) | Ovulation pain (mittelschmerz) |
| Dolore pulsante | Pulsing pain |
| Dolore pungente | Twinging pain |
| Dolore tagliente | Sharp pain |
| Dolore toracico | Chest pain |
| Dotto arterioso di Botallo | Ductus arteriosus (ductus Botalli shunt) |
| Dotto arterioso persistente (ductus arteriosus persistente) | Patent ductus arteriosus (persistent ductus arteriosus) |
| Dracunculiasi | Dracunculiasis |
| Ebola | Ebola hemorrhagic fever |
| Eccessiva crescita della lingua (macroglossia) | Enlarged tongue (macroglossia) |
| Eccesso di colesterolo nel sangue (ipercolesterolemia) | High blood cholesterol (hypercholesterolemia) |
| Eccesso di glucosio nel sangue (iperglicemia) | High blood sugar (hyperglicemia) |
| Echinococcosi (idatidosi) | Echinococcosis (hydatid disease) |
| Echinococcosi epatica | Hepatic echinococcosis |
| Echinococcosi polmonare | Pulmonary echinococcosis |
| Ecolalia | Echolalia |
| Ecoprassia (imitazione spontanea di movimenti osservati) | Echopraxia (involuntary repetition of the observed movements of another) |
| Eczema | Eczema |
| Edema | Edema |
| Edema cerebrale | Cerebral edema |
| Edema diffuso (anasarca) | Generalized edema (anasarca) |
| Edema polmonare | Pulmonary edema |
| Edema posturale | Postural edema |
| Eiaculazione precoce | Premature ejaculation |
| Elefantiasi | Elephantiasis (lymphedema) |
| Elettrosensibilità | Electromagnetic hypersensitivity |
| Elevata pressione intracranica | Intracranial hypertension |
| Emangioendotelioma | Hemangioendothelioma |
| Emangioma | Hemangioma |
| Emangioma capillare | Capillary hemangioma (infantile hemangioma, strawberry hemangioma) |
| Emangioma cavernoso | Cavernous hemangioma |
| Emartro | Bleeding into joint space (hemarthrosis) |
| Ematoma | Hematoma |
| Ematoma cerebrale | Intracerebral hematoma |
| Ematoma epidurale | Epidural hematoma |
| Ematoma subdurale | Subdural hematoma |
| Ematuria | Blood in urine (hematuria) |
| Embolia adiposa | Fat embolism |
| Embolia dell'arteria | Arterial embolism |
| Embolia gassosa | Air embolism (gas embolism) |
| Embolia polmonare | Pulmonary embolism |
| Embolismo (embolia) | Embolism |
| Emeralopia | Day blindness (hemeralopia) |
| Emesi emorragica (ematemesi) | Vomiting of blood (hematemesis) |
| Emicrania | Migraine |
| Emicrania cronica parossistica | Chronic paroxysmal hemicrania (Sjaastad syndrome) |
| Emissione di urine con difficoltà (disuria) | Difficult urination (dysuria) |
| Emivertebra | Hemivertebrae |
| Emocromatosi | Hemochromatosis |
| Emofilia | Hemophilia |
| Emopneumotorace | Hemopneumothorax |
| Emorragia | Bleeding (haemorrhage) |
| Emorragia arteriosa | Arterial bleeding |
| Emorragia cerebrale | Intracerebral hemorrhage |
| Emorragia epidurale | Epidural bleeding |
| Emorragia esterna | External bleeding |
| Emorragia interna | Internal bleeding |
| Emorragia subaracnoidea | Subarachnoid hemorrhage |
| Emorragia subdurale | Subdural hemorrhage |
| Emorragia venosa | Venous bleeding |

| | |
|---|---|
| Emorroidi | Hemorrhoids |
| Emosiderosi | Hemosiderosis |
| Emotorace | Hemothorax |
| Empiema | Empyema |
| Encefalite trasmessa da zecche | Tick-borne meningoencephalitis |
| Encefalocele | Encephalocele |
| Encefalopatia | Encephalopathy |
| Encondroma | Enchondroma |
| Enconpresi | Encopresis |
| Endocardite batterica | Bacterial endocarditis |
| Endometriosi | Endometriosis |
| Enfisema | Emphysema |
| Enfisema sottocutaneo | Subcutaneous emphysema |
| Entesopatia | Enthesopathy |
| Eosinofilia | Eosinophilia |
| Epatite virale | Viral hepatitis |
| Epatite virale A | Hepatitis A |
| Epatite virale B | Hepatitis B |
| Epatite virale C | Hepatitis C |
| Epatite virale D | Hepatitis D |
| Epatite virale E | Hepatitis E |
| Ependimoma | Ependymoma |
| Epifisiolisi della testa femorale | Epiphyseolysis capitis femoris |
| Epilessia | Epilepsy |
| Epispadia | Epispadias |
| Epistassi (rinorragia) | Nose bleeding (epistaxis) |
| Erezione persistente dolorosa (priapismo) | Long-lasting painful erection (priapism) |
| Erisipela | Erysipelas (Ignis sacer, St. Anthony's fire) |
| Erisipeloide | Erysipeloid |
| Eritema | Redness of the skin (erythema) |
| Eritema infettivo (quinta malattia) | Infectious erythema (fifth disease) |
| Eritroblastosi fetale (malattia emolitica del neonato) | Rh incompatibility (hemolytic disease of the newborn) |
| Eritromelalgia | Erythromelalgia (acromelalgia) |
| Eritroplachia (eritroplasia) | Erythroplakia (erythroplasia) |
| Eritroplasia di Queyrat | Erythroplasia of Queyrat |
| Ermafroditismo | Hermaphroditism |
| Ernia | Hernia |
| Ernia del disco | Spinal disc herniation |
| Ernia diaframmatica | Diaphragmatic hernia |
| Ernia esterna addominale | External abdominal wall hernia |
| Ernia iatale | Hiatus hernia |
| Ernia inguinale | Inguinal hernia |
| Ernia ombelicale | Umbilical hernia |
| Erosione cervicale | Cervical erosion |
| Erpangina (faringite vescicolare) | Herpangina (mouth blisters) |
| Eruttazione | Burping (belching) |
| Esantema | Exanthem |
| Esasperazione (irritazione) | Exasperation |
| Esoftalmo | Bulging eyes (exophthalmos) |
| Esostosi | Exostosis |
| Esostosi multipla ereditaria | Hereditary multiple exostoses |
| Espettorazione di sangue (emottisi) | Expectoration of blood (hemoptysis) |
| Esposizione alle radiazioni ionizzanti | Ionising irradiation |
| Fame | Hunger |
| Fame d'aria (dispnea, respirazione difficoltosa) | Shortness of breath (dyspnea) |
| Faringite streptococcica | Streptococcal pharyngitis |
| Fasciosi plantare | Plantar fasciitis |
| Fascite necrotizzante | Necrotizing fasciitis |
| Febbre | Fever |
| Febbre da fieno | Farmer's lung |
| Febbre da inalazione di fumi metallici | Metal fume fever |
| Febbre da morso di ratto | Rat-bite fever |
| Febbre da pappataci (febbre da Flebotomi) | Pappataci fever (phlebotomus fever, sandfly fever) |
| Febbre da zecca del Colorado | Colorado tick fever (mountain tick fever) |
| Febbre del Nilo occidentale | West Nile fever |
| Febbre della Rift Valley | Rift Valley fever |
| Febbre di Lassa | Lassa fever |
| Febbre di Oroya | Oroya fever (Carrion's disease) |
| Febbre emorragica | Viral hemorrhagic fever |
| Febbre emorragica con sindrome renale (febbre emorragica coreana) | Hemorrhagic fever with renal syndrome (Korean hemorrhagic fever) |
| Febbre emorragica Crimean-Congo | Crimean-Congo hemorrhagic fever |
| Febbre emorragica di Marburg | Marburg hemorrhagic fever |
| Febbre gialla | Yellow fever |
| Febbre mediterranea familiare | Familial Mediterranean fever |
| Febbre paratifoide | Paratyphoid fever |

| | |
|---|---|
| Febbre Q | Q fever |
| Febbre reumatica | Rheumatic fever |
| Febbre ricorrente | Relapsing fever |
| Febbre tifoide (tifo) | Typhoid fever (typhoid) |
| Febbre Zika | Zika fever |
| Feci di colore rosso | Red colored stool |
| Feci di colore verde | Green stool |
| Feci gialle | Yellow stool |
| Feci picee (melena) | Black stool (melena) |
| Fenilchetonuria | Phenylketonuria |
| Fenomeno di Bell | Bell's phenomenon |
| Feocromocitoma | Pheochromocytoma |
| Ferita | Wound (injury, lesion) |
| Ferita chimica | Chemical injuries |
| Ferita da arma da fuoco | Gunshot wound |
| Ferita da morso | Bite wound |
| Ferita da punta | Stab wound |
| Ferita da taglio | Cut wound |
| Ferita esplosiva | Explosive wound |
| Ferita termica | Thermal wound |
| Ferite provocate da esplosioni termonucleari | Thermonuclear injuries |
| Fibrillazione atriale | Atrial fibrillation |
| Fibrillazione ventricolare | Ventricular fibrillation |
| Fibroadenoma | Fibroadenoma |
| Fibroelastosi endocardica | Endocardial fibroelastosis |
| Fibroistiocitoma benigno | Fibrous histiocytoma |
| Fibroma | Fibroma |
| Fibroma condromixoide | Chondromyxoid fibroma |
| Fibromialgia | Fibromyalgia |
| Fibrosarcoma | Fibrosarcoma (fibroblastic sarcoma) |
| Fibrosi | Fibrosis |
| Fibrosi cistica | Cystic fibrosis |
| Fibrosi polmonare idiopatica | Idiopathic pulmonary fibrosis |
| Fibrosi retroperitoneale | Retroperitoneal fibrosis (Ormond's disease) |
| Fibrosi tendinea | Tendinous fibrositis |
| Fibrosite di mano | Hand fibrositis |
| Fibrosite muscolare | Muscular fibrositis |
| Filariasi | Filariasis |
| Fimosi | Phimosis |
| Fissura anale | Anal fissure |
| Fistola | Fistula |
| Fistola anale | Anal fistula |
| Fistola broncopleurica | Bronchopleural fistula |
| Flebotrombosi | Phlebothrombosis |
| Flemmone | Phlegmon |
| Flusso di sangue nella tuba di Falloppio | Bleeding into the fallopian tube (hematosalpinx) |
| Fobia | Phobia |
| Folgorazione (elettrocuzione) | Electrical injuries (electric shock) |
| Follicolite | Folliculitis |
| Follicoloma | Granulosa cell tumor |
| Forfora | Dandruff |
| Foruncolo | Furuncle (boil) |
| Fotofobia | Photophobia (fear of light) |
| Framboesia | Yaws (pian) |
| Frattura | Broken bone (bone fracture) |
| Frattura a legno verde | Greenstick fracture |
| Frattura a spirale | Spiral fracture |
| Frattura aperta (frattura esposta) | Open fracture (compound fracture) |
| Frattura comminuta | Comminuted fracture |
| Frattura con dislocazione | Fracture with displacement |
| Frattura da stress | Stress fracture |
| Frattura da stress della tibia | Tibia stress fracture |
| Frattura del bacino | Broken pelvis (pelvis fracture) |
| Frattura del calcagno | Broken heel bone (calcaneus fracture) |
| Frattura del capitello radiale | Radial head fracture (radial capitulum fracture) |
| Frattura del collo del femore | Femoral neck fracture |
| Frattura del collo dell'omero | Humeral neck fracture |
| Frattura del corpo vertebrale | Broken vertebral body (vertebral corpus fracture) |
| Frattura del femore | Broken thighbone (femur fracture) |
| Frattura del metatarso | Broken foot (metatarsal fracture) |
| Frattura del radio | Radius fracture |
| Frattura del terzo distale di tibia e perone | Supramaleolar fracture of tibia and fibula |
| Frattura dell'alluce | Broken big toe (fractured hallux) |
| Frattura dell'epicondilo omerale | Epicondylar elbow fracture |
| Frattura dell'olecrano | Broken elbow (olecranon fracture) |
| Frattura dell'omero | Broken upper arm (humerus fracture) |
| Frattura dell'osso navicolare | Broken navicular bone (navicular fracture) |

| | |
|---|---|
| Frattura dell'ulna | Broken ulna (ulna fracture) |
| Frattura della base del cranio | Base of skull fracture (basal skull fracture) |
| Frattura della caviglia | Broken ankle (ankle fracture) |
| Frattura della clavicola | Broken collarbone (clavicle fracture) |
| Frattura della costola | Broken rib (rib fracture) |
| Frattura della diafisi femorale | Diaphyseal tightbone fracture |
| Frattura della falange del dito | Broken finger (finger fracture) |
| Frattura della fibula | Broken fibula (fibula fracture) |
| Frattura della mascella e/o della mandibola | Upper and/or lower jaw fracture (broken upper/lower jaw) |
| Frattura della rotula | Broken knee cap (patellar fracture) |
| Frattura della scapola | Broken shoulder blade (scapula fracture) |
| Frattura della tibia | Broken shinbone (tibia fracture) |
| Frattura di Pouteau-Colles (frattura delle metafisi radiali distali) | Distal radial fracture |
| Frattura di radio e ulna | Broken forearm (fractured ulna and radius) |
| Frattura di tibia e perone | Broken lower leg bones (fractured tibia and fibula) |
| Frattura diafisaria dell'omero | Diaphyseal humeral fracture |
| Frattura incompleta (infrazione) | Incomplete fracture |
| Frattura obliqua | Oblique fracture |
| Frattura ripetuta | Refracturing (repeated fracture) |
| Frattura semplice | Simple bone fracture |
| Frattura sovracondiloidea del femore | Supracondylar femoral fracture |
| Frattura sovracondiloidea di omero | Supracondylar humerus fracture |
| Frattura trasversale | Transverse fracture |
| Fratture spontanee | Spontaneous fractures |
| Frigidità | Frigidity |
| Fuoriuscita (scolo) | Discharge |
| Fuoriuscita di sangue dall'orecchio (otorragia) | Ear bleeding |
| Fuoriuscita vaginale | Vaginal discharge |
| Fusione di vertebre cervicali (Sindrome di Klippel Feil) | Congenital fusion of cervical vertebrae (Klippel-Feil syndrome) |
| Galattorrea | Galactorrhea |
| Gangrena di Fournier | Fournier gangrene |
| Gangrena secca | Dry gangrene |
| Gangrena umida | Wet gangrene |
| Gangrene gassosa | Gas gangrene |
| Gastralgia | Epigastric pain |
| Gastroenterite | Gastroenteritis |
| Giardiasi (lambliasi) | Lambliasis (giardiasis) |
| Gibbo (gobba, gibbosità) | Hunchback |
| Gigantismo | Gigantism |
| Ginecomastia | Gynecomastia |
| Ginocchio del nuotatore a rana (stiramento cronico del legamento mediale) | Swimmer's knee |
| Ginocchio valgo | Knock knees (genu valgum) |
| Ginocchio varo (genu varum) | Bow legs (genu varum) |
| Giocco d'azzardo patologico | Gambling addiction (ludomania) |
| Glaucoma | Glaucoma |
| Glicosuria (mellituria) | Glucose in urine (glycosuria) |
| Glioblastoma | Glioblastoma |
| Glioma | Glioma |
| Gliosi | Gliosis |
| Glomangioma (paraganglioma) | Glomus tumor (glomangioma) |
| Glomerulonefrite | Glomerulonephritis |
| Gomito del tennista (epicondilite) | Tennis elbow |
| Gonadoblastoma | Gonadoblastoma |
| Gonfiezza e venti (flatulenza) | Bloating and gases (flatulence) |
| Gonfiore | Swelling |
| Gonorrea (blenorragia) | Gonorrhea |
| Gotta | Gout (gouty arthritis) |
| Gozzo | Goiter |
| Gozzo multinodulare | Nodular goiter |
| Graffio (graffiatura) | Scratch |
| Granulocitosi | Granulocytosis |
| Gravidanza ectopica | Ectopic pregnancy (extrauterine pregnancy) |
| Herpes genitalis | Genital herpes |
| Herpes simplex | Herpes simplex |
| Herpes zoster | Herpes zoster |
| Ictus emorragico | Hemorrhagic brain infarction |
| Idremia | Hydremia |

| | |
|---|---|
| Idrocefalo | Hydrocephalus |
| Idrocele | Hydrocele |
| Idrofobia | Aquaphobia |
| Idronefrosi | Hydronephrosis |
| Idrope | Hydrops |
| Idrope della colecisti | Gallbladder hydrops |
| Idropericardio | Pericardial effusion (hydropericard) |
| Idrotorace | Hydrothorax |
| Ifema | Hyphema |
| Igroma | Hygroma |
| Ileo | Ileus |
| Imbecillità | Imbecility |
| Immunodeficienza | Immunodeficiency |
| Impetigine | Impetigo |
| Impotenza | Impotency |
| Impulso a vomitare | Urge to vomit |
| Incapacità di percipire gli odori (disosmia) | Loss of olfaction (anosmia) |
| Incapacità di percipire i sapori (ageusia) | Loss of the sense of taste (ageusia) |
| Incontinenza | Incontinence |
| Incontinenza urinaria | Urinary incontinence |
| Incontinenza urinaria da sforzo | Stress urinary incontinence |
| Incoscienza (stato di incoscienza) | Unconsciousness |
| Indigestione | Indigestion |
| Induratio penis plastica (malattia di Peyronie) | Peyronie's disease (induratio penis plastica) |
| Inedia | Starvation |
| Infarto | Infarct |
| Infarto miocardico acuto | Heart attack (myocardial infarction) |
| Infarto polmonare | Pulmonary infarction |
| Infestazione da pidocchi (pediculosi) | Infestation with head lice (pediculosis) |
| Infestazione da pidocchi del pube (ftiriasi) | Infestation with pubic lice (phthiriasis) |
| Infestazione da vermi (elmintiasi) | Infestation with intestinal parasitic warms (helminthiasis) |
| Infezione (malattia infettiva) | Infection |
| Infezione batterica | Bacterial infection |
| Infezione da clamidia | Chlamydia infection |
| Infezione da Papilloma Virus Umano (HPV) | Human papilloma virus (HPV) infection |
| Infezione del tratto respiratorio superiore | Upper respiratory tract infection |
| Infezione dell'apparato osteo-articolare (osteomielite) | Infection of the bone or bone marrow (osteomyelitis) |
| Infezione della vagina batterica (vaginosi) | Bacterial vaginosis |
| Infezione fungina | Fungal infection |
| Infezione virale | Viral infection |
| Infiammazione (flogosi) | Inflammation |
| Infiammazione articolare (artrite) | Inflammation of the joint (arthritis) |
| Infiammazione dei bronchi (bronchite) | Inflammation of the bronchi (bronchitis) |
| Infiammazione dei bronchioli (bronchiolite) | Inflammation of the bronchioles (bronchiolitis) |
| Infiammazione dei polmoni (polmonite) | Inflammation of the lung (pneumonia) |
| Infiammazione dei reni (nefrite) | Inflammation of the kidney (nephritis) |
| Infiammazione dei seni paranasali (sinusite) | Inflammation of the paranasal sinuses (sinusitis) |
| Infiammazione dei tessuti gengivali (gengivite) | Inflammation of the gums (gingivitis) |
| Infiammazione dei testicoli (orchite) | Inflammation of the testes (orchitis) |
| Infiammazione del cervello (encefalite) | Inflammation of the brain (encephalitis) |
| Infiammazione del fegato (epatite) | Inflammation of the liver (hepatitis) |
| Infiammazione del miocardio (miocardite) | Inflammation of the heart muscle (myocarditis) |
| Infiammazione del nervo (neurite, nevrite) | Inflammation of the nerve (neuritis) |
| Infiammazione del pancreas (pancreatite) | Inflammation of the pancreas (pancreatitis) |
| Infiammazione del parametrio (parametrite) | Inflammation of the parametrium (parametritis) |
| Infiammazione del pericardio (pericardite) | Inflammation of the pericardium (pericarditis) |
| Infiammazione del tendine (tendinite) | Inflammation of the tendon (tendinitis, tendonitis) |
| Infiammazione del tessuto muscolare (miosite) | Inflammation of the muscles (myositis) |
| Infiammazione del timo | Inflammation of the thymus (thymitis) |
| Infiammazione dell'epiglottide (epiglottite) | Inflammation of the epiglottis (epiglottitis) |

| | |
|---|---|
| Infiammazione dell'appendice vermiforme (appendicite) | Inflammation of the appendix (appendicitis) |
| Infiammazione dell'endocardio (endocardite) | Inflammation of the endocardium (endocarditis) |
| Infiammazione dell'endometrio (endometrite) | Inflammation of the endometrium (endometritis) |
| Infiammazione dell'epididimo (epididimite) | Inflammation of the epididymis (epididymitis) |
| Infiammazione dell'inserzione di muscolo (entesite) | Inflammation of the entheses (enthesitis) |
| Infiammazione dell'uretra (uretrite) | Inflammation of the urethra (urethritis) |
| Infiammazione della borsa sierosa di un'articolazione (borsite) | Inflammation of the synovial fluid sac (bursitis) |
| Infiammazione della colecisti (colecistite) | Inflammation of the gall bladder (cholecystitis) |
| Infiammazione della congiuntiva (congiuntivite) | Inflammation of the conjunctiva (conjunctivitis) |
| Infiammazione della cornea (cheratite) | Inflammation of the cornea (keratitis) |
| Infiammazione della cornea e della congiutiva (cherato-tocongiuntivite) | Inflammation of the cornea and conjunctiva (kerato-conjunctivitis) |
| Infiammazione della fascia (fascite) | Inflammation of the fascia (fasciitis) |
| Infiammazione della ghiandola prostatica (prostatite) | Inflammation of the prostate gland (prostatitis) |
| Infiammazione della laringe (laringite) | Inflammation of the larynx (laryngitis) |
| Infiammazione della mammella (mastite) | Inflammation of the breast (mastitis) |
| Infiammazione della membrana sinoviale (sinovite) | Inflammation of the synovial membrane (synovitis) |
| Infiammazione della mucosa gastrica (gastrite) | Inflammation of the stomach lining (gastritis) |
| Infiammazione della pelle (dermatite) | Inflammation of the skin (dermatitis) |
| Infiammazione della pleura (pleurite) | Inflammation of the pleura (pleuritis) |
| Infiammazione della retina (retinite) | Inflammation of the retina (retinitis) |
| Infiammazione della sierosa peritoneale (peritonite) | Inflammation of the peritoneum (peritonitis) |
| Infiammazione della testa del glande (balanite) | Inflammation of the glans penis (balanitis) |
| Infiammazione della tiroide (tiroidite) | Inflammation of the thyroid gland (thyroiditis) |
| Infiammazione della trachea (tracheite) | Inflammation of the windpipe (tracheitis) |
| Infiammazione della tunica media dell'occhio (uveite) | Inflammation of the middle layer of the eye (uveitis) |
| Infiammazione della vagina (vaginite) | Inflammation of the vagina (vaginitis) |
| Infiammazione della vescica urinaria (cistite) | Inflammation of the urinary bladder (cystitis) |
| Infiammazione della vulva (vulvite) | Inflammation of the vulva (vulvitis) |
| Infiammazione delle arterie (arterite) | Inflammation of the arterial walls (arteritis) |
| Infiammazione delle ghiandole linfatiche (linfoadenite) | Inflammation of the lymph node (lymphadenitis) |
| Infiammazione delle ghiandole salivari (sialoadenite) | Inflammation of the salivary gland (sialadenitis) |
| Infiammazione delle meningi (meningite) | Inflammation of the meninges (meningitis) |
| Infiammazione delle mucose della bocca (stomatite) | Inflammation of the mouth mucous lining (stomatitis) |
| Infiammazione delle tonsille (tonsillite) | Inflammation of the tonsils (tonsillitis) |
| Infiammazione delle vene (flebite) | Inflammation of the vein (phlebitis) |
| Infiammazione di labirinto nell'orecchio interno (labirintite) | Inflammation of the inner ear (labyrinthitis) |
| Infiammazione di tendine e di guaina tendinea (tenosinovite) | Inflammation of the synovium and tendon (tenosynovitis) |
| Infiammazione granulomatosa | Granulomatous inflammation |
| Influenza | Flu (influenza) |
| Influenza aviaria H5N1 | Bird flu (influenzavirus A subtype H5N1) |
| Influenza spagnola | Spanish flu |

| | |
|---|---|
| Influenza suina | Pig flu (swine influenza, influenzavirus A subtype H1N1) |
| Infreddatura (raffreddore) | Common cold |
| Ingrossamento (divenire grosso) | Gaining weight |
| Ingrossamento dei linfonodi (linfoadenopatia) | Enlarged lymph nodes (lymphadenopathy) |
| Insolazione (colpo di sole) | Sunstroke (heat stroke) |
| Insonnia | Insomnia |
| Insufficienza epatica | Liver insufficiency |
| Insufficienza renale | Kidney failure (renal insufficiency) |
| Insufficienza renale acuta | Acute kidney failure |
| Insufficienza renale cronica | Chronic renal failure |
| Insufficienza venosa cronica cerebrospinale | Chronic cerebrospinal venous insufficiency |
| Intolleranza al glutine | Gluten intolerance |
| Intolleranza al lattosio | Lactose intolerance |
| Intormentire | Tingling |
| Intossicazione alimentare da stafilococco | Staphylococcal food poisoning |
| Intossicazione da metalli pesanti | Heavy metal poisoning |
| Iperaldosteronismo | Aldosteronism (hyperaldosteronism) |
| Iperattività | Hyperactivity |
| Ipercalcemia | Hypercalcemia |
| Iperestenzione della regione posteriore del tronco (opistotono) | Spastic arching position (opisthotonus) |
| Iperinsulinismo | Hyperinsulinism |
| Iperkaliemia | Hyperkalemia |
| Ipermetropia | Farsightedness (hyperopia) |
| Iperparatiroidismo | Hyperparathyroidism |
| Iperpituitarismo | Hyperpituitarism |
| Iperplasia endometriale | Endometrial hyperplasia |
| Iperplasia pseudo-epiteliomatosa | Pseudoepitheliomatous hyperplasia |
| Ipertensione arteriosa essenziale | Essential hypertension |
| Ipertensione arteriosa polmonare | Pulmonary hypertension |
| Ipertensione arteriosa secondaria | Secondary hypertension (inessential hypertension) |
| Ipertensione arteriosa sistemica | High blood pressure (hypertension) |
| Ipertensione maligna | Malignant hypertension |
| Ipertensione portale | Portal hypertension |
| Ipertensione renale | Renovacsular hypertension |
| Ipertermia | Hyperthermia |
| Ipertiroidismo | Hyperthyroidism |
| Ipertrofia | Hypertrophy |
| Ipertrofia prostatica benigna | Benign prostatic hyperthroph |
| Ipertrofia ventricolare | Ventricular hypertrophy |
| Iperuricemia | Hyperuricemia |
| Iperventilazione | Hyperventilation |
| Ipervitaminosi | Hypervitaminosis |
| Ipervolemia (aumento del volume ematico circolante) | Hypervolemia (increased level of fluid in the blood) |
| Ipoalbuminemia | Hypoalbuminemia |
| Ipocalcemia | Hypocalcemia |
| Ipocondria | Hypochondria |
| Ipoglicemia | Hypoglycemia |
| Ipoinsulinemia | Hypoinsulinism |
| Ipokaliemia | Hypokalemia |
| Ipoparatiroidismo | Hypoparathyroidism |
| Ipopituitarismo | Hypopituitarism |
| Ipoplasia del tronco polmonare | Pulmonary hypoplasia |
| Ipospadia | Hypospadias |
| Ipossia | Hypoxia |
| Ipotensione e sincope | Hypotension and syncope |
| Ipotermia | Hypothermia |
| Ipotiroidismo | Hypothyroidism |
| Ipotonia | Hypotonia |
| Ipotonia muscolare | Muscular hypotonia |
| Ippersensibilità ai normali stimoli esterni (iperestesia) | Increased sensitivity to stimuli of the senses (hyperesthesia) |
| Iridodialisi | Iridodialysis (coredialysis) |
| Irite | Iritis |
| Irradiazione non ionizzante | Non-ionising irradiation |
| Irradiazione radioattiva | Radioactive irradiation |
| Irsutismo | Hirsutism |
| Ischemia | Ischemia |
| Ischemia degli arti | Ischemic limbs |
| Ischemia miocardica | Ischemic heart disease |
| Isosporiasi | Isosporiasis |
| Isteria (isterismo) | Hysteria |
| Istoplasmosi | Histoplasmosis (Darling's disease) |
| Ittero (itterizia) | Jaundice (icterus) |
| Ittero neonatale | Neonatal jaundice |

| | |
|---|---|
| Ittero ostruttivo | Mechanic icterus (bile duct obstruction) |
| Kala-azar (febbre d'Assam, splenomegalia infantile) | Kala-azar (black fever) |
| Kernittero (encefalopatia bilirubinica) | Kernicterus |
| Kuru | Kuru |
| Labbro leporino | Cleft lip and palate |
| Lacerazione (strappo) | Laceration (tear) |
| Lacerazione cerebrale | Brain laceration |
| Laringospasmo | Laryngospasm |
| Lebbra | Leprosy |
| Leiomioma | Leiomyoma |
| Leiomiosarcoma | Leiomyosarcoma |
| Leishmaniosi | Leishmaniasis |
| Leishmaniosi cutanea | Cutaneous leishmaniasis (Oriental sore) |
| Lentezza psicofisica | Slow psychophysiological responses |
| Leptospirosi | Leptospirosis |
| Lesione del nervo | Nerve lesion |
| Lesione del nervo periferico | Peripheral nerve lesion |
| Lesione ostruttiva dell'intestino tenue | Obstructive lesion of the small intestine |
| Lesioni da scoppio (blast-syndrome) | Blast-syndrome |
| Lesioni della testa e del cervello | Head and brain injuries |
| Lesioni meccaniche | Mechanical injuries |
| Lesioni termiche | Thermal injuries |
| Leucemia | Leukemia |
| Leucemia acuta linfoblastica | Acute lymphoblastic leukemia |
| Leucemia linfatica | Lymphatic leukemia |
| Leucemia linfatica cronica | Chronic lymphocytic leukemia |
| Leucemia mieloide | Myeloid leukemia |
| Leucemia mieloide acuta | Acute myeloid leukemia (AML) |
| Leucemia mieloide cronica | Chronic myeloid leukemia |
| Leucemia monocitica | Monocytic leukemia |
| Leucocitosi | Leukocytosis |
| Leucodistrofia | Leukodystrophy |
| Leucoplachia | Leukoplakia |
| Leucorea | Leukorrhea |
| Lichen planus | Lichen planus |
| Linfadenite tubercolare | Tuberculous lymphadenitis |
| Linfangioma | Lymphangioma |
| Linfangiosarcoma | Lymphangiosarcoma |
| Linfedema | Lymphedema |
| Linfoma | Lymphoma |
| Linfoma di Hodgkin | Hodgkin's disease |
| Linfoma non Hodgkin | Non-Hodgkin's lymphoma |
| Lipodistrofia | Lipodystrophy |
| Lipoma | Lipoma |
| Lipomatosi pancreatica | Pancreatic lipomatosis |
| Liposarcoma | Liposarcoma |
| Listeriosi | Listeriosis |
| Lobster-claw deformità di piede | Split foot (lobster claw foot, ectrodactyly) |
| Lombaggine | Low back pain (lumbago, lumbosacral syndrome) |
| Lombalgia dell'atleta | Gymnastics lower back pain |
| Lordosi | Lordosis |
| Lupus eritematoso sistemico | Lupus erythematosus |
| Lussazione | Dislocation (luxation) |
| Lussazione acromio-clavicolare | Separated shoulder (acromi-oclavicular dislocation) |
| Lussazione congenita dell'anca (displasia dell'anca) | Congenital dysplasia of the hip (congenital hip dislocation) |
| Lussazione del ginocchio | Knee dislocation (luxation of the knee) |
| Lussazione del gomito | Elbow dislocation (luxation of the elbow) |
| Lussazione dell'anca | Dislocation of a hip |
| Lussazione della caviglia | Dislocated ankle joint |
| Lussazione della mandibola | Mandibular dislocation |
| Lussazione della rotula | Luxating patella (trick knee, floating patella) |
| Lussazione della spalla | Dislocated shoulder |
| Lussazione incompleta (sublussazione) | Partial dislocation (subluxation) |
| Lussazioni delle atricolazioni della mano e delle dita | Hand and finger joints dislocation |
| Macchie di Koplik | Koplik's spots |
| Mal di denti | Toothache |
| Mal di gola (infiammazione della faringe, faringite) | Sore throat (inflammation of the throat, pharyngitis) |
| Mal di mare | Seasickness |

| | |
|---|---|
| Mal di montagna | Altitude sickness (acute mountain sickness) |
| Mal di schiena (dorsopatia) | Back pain (dorsalgia) |
| Mal di schiena su base posturale | Postural back pain |
| Mal di testa | Headache |
| Malaria | Malaria |
| Malassorbimento | Malabsorption |
| Malattia autoimmunitaria | Autoimmune disease |
| Malattia da vibrazioni | Vibration disease |
| Malattia dei riempitori dei silos | Silo-filler's disease |
| Malattia del cuore (cardiopatia) | Heart disease (cardiopathy) |
| Malattia del motoneurone | Motor neurone disease |
| Malattia di Bornholm (mialgia epidemica) | Bornholm disease (epidemic myalgia) |
| Malattia di Brill-Zinsser | Brill's disease |
| Malattia di Chagas | Chagas disease (American trypanosomiasis) |
| Malattia di Charcot-Marie-Tooth | Charcot-Marie-Tooth disease |
| Malattia di Creutzfeldt-Jakob (cosiddetta "malattia della mucca pazza") | Creutzfeldt-Jakob disease (so called "mad cow disease") |
| Malattia di Crohn | Crohn's disease |
| Malattia di decompressione (sindrome di Caisson) | Decompression sickness (diver's disease, caisson disease) |
| Malattia di Dupuytren | Dupuytren's contracture |
| Malattia di Freiberg | Freiberg's disease |
| Malattia di Haglund (deformità di Haglund) | Haglund's disease |
| Malattia di Hirschsprung (malattia di Mya) | Hirschsprung's disease (congenital aganglionic megacolon) |
| Malattia di Huntington | Huntington's chorea (Huntington's disease) |
| Malattia di Köhler | Köhler disease |
| Malattia di Legg-Perthes-Calvé | Legg-Calvé-Perthes disease |
| Malattia di Lyme (borreliosi di Lyme) | Lyme disease (lyme borreliosis) |
| Malattia di Morquio (mucopolisaccaridosi IV) | Morquio's syndrome (mucopolysaccharidosis IV) |
| Malattia di Panner | Panner's disease |
| Malattia di Pellegrini-Stieda | Pellegrini-Stieda disease |
| Malattia di Sever | Sever's disease |
| Malattia di Van Neck | Van Neck disease |
| Malattia infiammatoria pelvica | Pelvic inflammatory disease |
| Malattia parassitaria (parassitosi) | Parasitic disease (parasitosis) |
| Malattia professionale | Occupational disease |
| Malattia sessualmente trasmissibile | Sexually transmitted disease |
| Malattie dei vasi sanguigni | Blood vessel diseases |
| Malattie dell'aorta | Diseases of the aorta |
| Malattie delle valvole cardiache | Heart valve diseases |
| Malattie infettive dei bambini | Childhood infectious diseases |
| Mancanza dell'appetito | Loss of appetite |
| Mancanza di movimento | Movement inability |
| Mancata discesa del testicolo | Undescended testicle |
| Mancata secrezione di urina | Inability to urinate |
| Mancato sviluppo di un organo (aplasia di un organo) | Absence in development of an organ (aplasia of an organ) |
| Mania | Mania |
| Mastopatia | Mastopathy |
| Mastopatia fibrocistica | Fibrocystic breast disease |
| Medulloblastoma | Medulloblastoma |
| Megacolon | Megacolon |
| Melanoma | Melanoma |
| Melasma | Melasma (chloasma faciei) |
| Melioidosi | Melioidosis (Whitmore disease) |
| Meningioma | Meningioma |
| Meningocele | Meningocele |
| Meningoencefalite amebica primaria | Primary amoebic meningoencephalitis |
| Meningoencefalocele | Meningoencephalocele |
| Meniscopatia | Meniscal disease |
| Menopausa | Menopause |
| Mesotelioma | Mesothelioma |
| Mesotelioma sarcomatoide | Sarcomatoid mesothelioma |

| | |
|---|---|
| Mestruazione dolorosa (dismenorrea) | Painful menstruation (dysmenorrhea) |
| Metabolismo basale accelerato | Accelerated basal metabolism |
| Metamorfosi grassa del fegato | Fatty liver metamorphosis |
| Metastasi | Metastasis |
| Metatarsalgia | Metatarsalgia (Morton's neuroma) |
| Meteoropatia | Meteoropathy |
| Mialgia cervicale | Neck myalgia |
| Miastenia gravis | Myasthenia gravis |
| Micetoma | Mycetoma |
| Micosi | Mycosis |
| Mieloma multiplo | Plasmacytoma (multiple myeloma) |
| Mielomeningocele | Meningomyelocele |
| Miliaria rubra | Miliaria rubra (sweat rash) |
| Minzione dolorosa (stranguria) | Painful urination (strangury) |
| Mioblastoma | Myoblastoma |
| Miocardiopatia alcolica | Alcoholic cardiomyopathy |
| Mioclono | Myoclonic twitches (myoclonus) |
| Miogelosi | Myogelosis |
| Mioma | Myoma |
| Miopia | Shortsightedness (myopia) |
| Miosarcoma | Myosarcoma |
| Miosite ossificante | Myositis ossificans |
| Miosite ossificante progressiva | Myositis ossificans progressiva |
| Miscela di gas (flatulenza) | Passing gas (flatulence, farting) |
| Mixedema | Myxedema |
| Mixoma | Myxoma |
| Mixosarcoma | Myxosarcoma |
| Mollusco contagioso | Molluscum contagiosum |
| Mollusco pendule (fibroma molle) | Soft fibroma (fibroma molle, acrochordon) |
| Mononucleosi infettiva (malattia del bacio) | Infectious mononucleosis (Pfeiffer's disease, kissing disease, glandular fever) |
| Morbillo | Measles |
| Morbo di Addison | Addison's disease |
| Morbo di Alzheimer | Alzheimer's diesase |
| Morbo di Basedow-Graves | Basedow Graves disease |
| Morbo di Bowen | Bowen's disease (squamous cell carcinoma in situ) |
| Morbo di Buerger | Buerger's disease (thromboangiitis obliterans) |
| Morbo di Kienböck | Kienböck's disease |
| Morbo di Paget | Paget's disease |
| Morbo di Parkinson | Parkinson's disease |
| Morbo di Whipple | Whipple's disease |
| Morsicatura | Bite |
| Morsicatura di animale rabbioso | Bite by rabies infected animal |
| Morsicatura di cane | Dog bite |
| Morsicatura di gatto | Cat bite |
| Morsicatura di ragno | Spider bite |
| Morsicatura di ratto | Rat bite |
| Morsicatura di serpenti | Snake bite |
| Morsicatura di uomo | Human bite |
| Morsicatura di zecca infetta | Infected tick bite |
| Morso della vedova nera | Black widow bite |
| Morte | Death |
| Morte naturale | Natural death |
| Morte violenta | Violent death |
| Morva umana | Glanders |
| Movimenti incontrollati degli occhi (opsoclono) | Uncontrolled eye movement (opsoclonus) |
| Movimento anormale | Abnormal flexibility |
| MSSA (MRSA) | MRSA |
| Muco nasale | Nasal secretion (mucus) |
| Muco nelle feci | Mucus in stool |
| Mucocele | Mucocele |
| Mucopolisaccaridosi | Mucopolysaccharidosis |
| Mughetto (moniliasi orale) | Thrush (oral candidiasis) |
| Muscolo flaccido | Flaccid muscle (untoned muscle) |
| Nanismo | Dwarfism (nanism) |
| Narcolessia | Narcolepsy |
| Naso che cola (rinorrea) | Runny nose (rinorrhea) |
| Nausea | Nausea |
| Necrosi | Necrosis |
| Necrosi fibrinoide | Fibrinoid necrosis |
| Nefrite interstiziale | Interstitial nephritis |
| Nefropatia diabetica | Diabetic nephropathy |
| Nefrosi | Nephrosis |
| Neoplasie del tratto urogenitale | Urogenital neoplasm |
| Neurinoma (Schwannoma) | Neurinoma |
| Neuroblastoma | Neuroblastoma |
| Neuroborreliosi | Neuroborreliosis |
| Neurodermite (dermatite atopica) | Atopic dermatitis |

| | |
|---|---|
| Neurofibromatosi di tipo 1 (malattia di von Recklinghausen) | Neurofibromatosis type1 (Von Recklinghausen's disease) |
| Neuroma | Neuroma |
| Neuroma dell'acustico | Acoustic neuroma |
| Neuropatia | Neuropathy |
| Neuropatia diabetica | Diabetic neuropathy |
| Nevralgia | Neuralgia |
| Nevralgia del nervo cranico | Cranial neuralgia |
| Nevralgia del trigemino | Trigeminal neuralgia |
| Nevralgia occipitale (nevralgia di Arnold) | Occipital neuralgia (Arnold's neuralgia) |
| Nevrastenia | Neurasthenia |
| Nevrosi | Neurosis |
| Nistagmo | Nystagmus |
| Nodo (nodulo) | Knot (lump) |
| Noduli di Bouchard | Bouchard's nodes |
| Noduli di Heberden | Heberden's nodes |
| Nodulo di Suor Maria Giuseppa | Sister Mary Joseph nodule |
| Obesità | Obesity |
| Occhi lacrimosi | Watery eyes |
| Occhi secchi (xeroftalmia) | Dry eyes (keratoconjuctivitis sicca) |
| Occlusione arteria retinica | Retinal artery occlusion |
| Odore sgradevole dell'alito (alitosi, bromopnea) | Bad breath (halitosis) |
| Oligodendroglioma | Oligodendroglioma |
| Oligomenorrea | Oligomenorrhea |
| Oncocercosi (cecità fluviale) | Onchocerciasis (river blindness) |
| Orticaria | Hives (urticaria) |
| Osteitis fibrosa cistica | Osteitis fibrosa cystica |
| Osteoartropatia ipertrofizzante (sindrome di Pierre Marie-Bamberger) | Hyperthropic osteoarthropaty (Pierre Marie-Bamberger syndrome) |
| Osteoclastoma (tumore a cellule giganti) | Gigantocellular tumor (osteoclastoma) |
| Osteocondrite dissecante | Juvenile osteochondrosis |
| Osteocondroma | Osteochondroma |
| Osteogenesi imperfetta | Osteogenesis imperfecta (brittle bone disease) |
| Osteoma | Osteoma |
| Osteomalacia | Osteomalacia |
| Osteomielite fungale | Fungal osteomyelitis |
| Osteomielite luetica | Luetic osteomyelitis |
| Osteopetrosi (malattia delle ossa di marmo) | Osteopetrosis (marble bone disease) |
| Osteoporosi | Osteoporosis |
| Osteosarcoma | Osteosarcoma |
| Osteosclerosi | Osteosclerosis |
| Ottusità alle estremità | Dullness in limbs |
| Overdose di droga | Drug overdose |
| Overdose di farmaci | Medication overdose |
| Pallore | Paleness (pallor) |
| Palmi delle mani caldi e sudati | Warm sweaty palms |
| Pancraes aberrante | Aberrant pancreas |
| Papilledema (edema del nervo ottico) | Optic nerve edema |
| Papilloma | Papilloma |
| Paracoccidioidimicosi (blastomicosi sudamericana) | Paracoccidioidomycosis (Brazilian blastomycosis) |
| Parafimosi | Paraphimosis |
| Paragonimiasi | Paragonimiasis |
| Paralisi | Paralysis |
| Paralisi cerebrale infantile | Cerebral palsy |
| Paralisi dei arti superiori e inferiori (quadriplegia) | Paralysis of all limbs and torso (quadriplegia, tetraplegia) |
| Paralisi di Bell | Bell's palsy |
| Paralisi di parte inferiore del corpo (paraplegia) | Paralysis of lower extremities (paraplegia) |
| Paralisi di una metà del corpo (emiplegia) | Paralysis of one half of a body (hemiplegia) |
| Paralisi di una parte di corpo simmetrica (diplegia) | Paralysis of symmetrical parts of the body (diplegia) |
| Paranoia | Paranoia |
| Paresi | Paresis |
| Parestesie delle estremità | Numbness in limbs |
| Parodontite | Periodontitis |
| Paronichia | Paronychia |
| Parotite (orecchioni) | Mumps (epidemic parotitis) |
| Patereccio | Whitlow (felon) |
| Pemfigo | Pemphigus |
| Perdita dell'udito dovuta all'avanzamento dell'età (presbiacusia) | Age-related hearing loss (presbycusis) |
| Perdita dello strato superiore della pelle (desquamazione) | Shedding of the skin (desquamation) |

| | |
|---|---|
| Perdita di abilità di produzione del linguaggio verbale (afasia) | Loss of language ability (aphasia) |
| Perdita di liquido cerebrospinale dal naso (rinoliquorrea) | Leakage of cerebrospinal fluid through the nose |
| Perdita di liquido cerebrospinale dall'orechio (otoliquorrea) | Leakage of cerebrospinal fluid through the ear |
| Perdita di memoria | Memory loss |
| Perdita di metà di campo visivo (emianopsia) | Loss of half of a field of vision (hemianopsia) |
| Perdita di polso | Absence of pulse |
| Perdita di sangue al di fuori della mestruazione (metrorragia) | Uterine bleeding (metrorrhagia) |
| Perdita di sangue dall'ano (rettoragia, proctorragia) | Anal bleeding |
| Perdita di senso di tocco | Loss of the sense of touch |
| Perdita di udito | Hearing loss |
| Perforazione del timpano | Perforated eardrum (tympanorrhexis) |
| Periostite tibiale (sindrome del muscolo tibiale posteriore) | Tibialis posterior syndrome |
| Peritendite rotulea (ginocchio del saltatore) | Irritated knee (jumper's knee, patellar tendinopathy) |
| Perniosi | Chilblain (perniosis) |
| Pertosse | Whooping cough (pertussis) |
| Peste (pestilenza) | Plague (pest) |
| Petecchia | Petechia |
| Petto carenato | Pigeon chest (pectus carinatum) |
| Piaga da decubito (decubito) | Bedsore (decubitus ulcer) |
| Piede calcaneo | Pes calcaneus |
| Piede cavo (pes cavus) | High arches (pes cavus) |
| Piede d'atleta (tinea pedis) | Athlete's foot (tinea pedis) |
| Piede equino | Dancer's foot (pes equinus) |
| Piede equino (talipes equinovarus) | Club foot (talipes equinovarus) |
| Piede piatto (pes planus) | Flat foot (pes planus) |
| Piede piatto valgo (pes valgus) | Pes valgus |
| Pielonefrite | Pyelonephritis (kidney infection) |
| Pilorospasmo | Pylorospasm |
| Pinta | Pinta |
| Pionefrosi | Pyonephrosis |
| Pipita | Agnail (hangnail) |
| Piromania | Pyromania |
| Pitiriasi versicolor (tinea versicolor) | Tinea versicolor (pityriasis versicolor, haole rot) |
| Placca (tartaro) | Dental plaque (dental tartar) |
| Pneumoconiosi | Pneumoconiosis |
| Pneumopatia interstiziale | Interstitial lung disease |
| Pneumotorace | Pneumothorax |
| Policitemia | Polycythemia |
| Polidattilia | Polydactyly |
| Polimialgia reumatica | Polymyalgia rheumatica |
| Polimiosite | Polymyositis |
| Poliomielite (polio, paralisi infantile) | Poliomyelitis (polio, infantile paralysis) |
| Polipo | Polyp |
| Polipo cervicale | Cervical polyp |
| Polipo del colon | Colon polyp |
| Polipo della corda vocale | Vocal chords polyp |
| Polipo endometriale | Endometrial polyp (uterine polyp) |
| Polipo nasale | Nasal polyp |
| Polmonite atipica | Atypical pneumonia |
| Polmonite batterica | Bacterial pneumonia |
| Polmonite da Pneumocisti | Pneumocystis pneumonia (pneumocystosis) |
| Polmonite virale | Viral pneumonia |
| Polso accelerato | Accelerated pulse rate |
| Porfiria | Porphyria |
| Porpora | Purpura |
| Porpora trombotica trombocitopenica | Thrombotic thrombocytopenic purpura |
| Prematuro sviluppo sessuale del sesso opposto | Premature sexual development of the opposite sex |
| Prematuro sviluppo sessuale dello stesso sesso | Premature sexual development of the same sex |
| Presbiopia (presbitismo) | Age-related long-sightedness (presbyopia) |
| Presenza di emoglobina nelle urine (emoglobinuria) | Hemoglobin in urine (hemoglobinuria) |
| Presenza di pus nelle urine (piuria) | Pus in urine (pyuria) |
| Presenza di pus nello sputo | Pus in sputum |
| Primo flusso mestruale (menarca) | First menstrual cycle (menarche) |
| Proctite | Proctitis |

| | |
|---|---|
| Produzione di pochi spermatozoi (oligospermia) | Low semen volume (oligospermia) |
| Produzione di saliva eccessiva (ipersalivazione) | Excessive secretion of saliva (hypersalivation) |
| Prolasso del retto | Rectal prolapse |
| Prolasso uterino | Uterine prolapse (fallen womb) |
| Proteinosi alveolare polmonare | Pulmonary alveolar proteinosis |
| Proteinuria | Proteinuria (presence of proteins in urine) |
| Prurito (pizzicore) | Itching |
| Psiconevrosi (nevrosi) | Psychoneurosis |
| Psicopatia | Psychopathy |
| Psicosi | Psychosis |
| Psicosi maniaco-depressiva | Bipolar disorder (manic-depressive psychosis) |
| Psittacosi (psittacornitosi) | Psittacosis (parrot fever) |
| Psoriasi | Psoriasis |
| Pubalgia dello sportivo | Groin pain syndrome |
| Pubertà precoce (pubertà prematura) | Precocious puberty (premature puberty) |
| Pubertà tardiva | Delayed puberty |
| Puntura di formiche | Ant sting |
| Puntura di scorpione | Scorpion sting |
| Puntura di zanzara infetta | Infected mosquito bite |
| Pupille costrette | Small pupils |
| Pupille dilatate | Enlarged pupils |
| Pus | Pus |
| Pustola | Pustule |
| R.S.I. (Repetitive Strain Injury) | Repetitive strain injury (cumulative trauma disorder) |
| Rabbia | Rabies |
| Rabdomioma | Rhabdomyoma |
| Rabdomiosarcoma | Rhabdomyosarcoma |
| Rachitismo | Rickets (rachitis) |
| Rachitismo renale | Renal rickets |
| Raucedine | Hoarseness |
| Rene a ferro di cavallo (fusione renale) | Horseshoe kidney (renal fusion) |
| Rene policistico | Polycystic kidney disease |
| Respirazione difficoltosa | Breathing difficulty |
| Respirazione superficiale | Shallow breathing |
| Respiro di Biot | Biot's respiration |
| Respiro di Cheyne-Stokes | Periodic breathing (Cheyne-Stokes respiration) |
| Respiro di Kussmaul | Kussmaul breathing |
| Reticoloendotelioma (reticolosarcoma) | Reticuloendothelial sarcoma |
| Retinite pigmentosa | Retinitis pigmentosa (retinal pigment epithelium dystrophy) |
| Retinopatia del prematuro | Retinopathy of prematurity (retrolental fibroplasia) |
| Retinopatia diabetica | Diabetic retinopathy |
| Retroflessione uterina | Retroverted uterus |
| Rettocolite ulcerosa | Ulcerative colitis |
| Reumatismo extra-articolare | Extrajoint rheumatism |
| Rickettsiosi | Rickettsiosis |
| Ridotta mobilità articolare | Limited joint mobility |
| Riduzione della forza muscolare (astenia) | Loss of strenght (asthenia) |
| Riduzione della frequenza cardiaca (bradicardia) | Slow pulse rate (bradycardia) |
| Riduzione della frequenza respiratoria (bradipnea) | Slow breathing rate (bradypnea) |
| Rigidità | Stiffness |
| Rigidità dell'articolazione | Joint stiffness |
| Rigidità nucale | Nuchal rigidity (stiff neck) |
| Rinite | Rhinitis |
| Rinite allergica | Allergic rhinitis |
| Rinite vasomotoria | Vasomotor rhinitis |
| Ripugnanza al cibo | Food aversion |
| Risalita di alimenti dallo stomaco alla bocca (rigurgito) | Expulsion of undigested food from the mouth (regurgitation) |
| Ritardo mentale | Mental retardation |
| Ritenzione urinaria | Urinary retention (ischuria) |
| Rizartrosi (artrosi dell'articolazione alla base del police) | Thumb joint arthritis |
| Ronzio auricolare (acufene, tinnito) | Ringing in ears (tinnitus) |
| Rosacea | Rosacea |
| Rosolia | German measles (rubella) |
| Rottura | Rupture |
| Rottura del legamento | Ligament rupture (torn ligament) |

| | |
|---|---|
| Rottura del legamento crociato anteriore del ginocchio | Anterior cruciate ligament rupture (ACL rupture) |
| Rottura del menisco | Meniscus rupture (meniscus tear) |
| Rottura del tendine | Tendon rupture (torn tendon) |
| Rottura del tendine di Achille | Achilles tendon rupture |
| Rottura della cuffia dei rotatori | Rotator cuff rupture (rotator cuff tear) |
| Rottura della milza | Ruptured spleen |
| Rottura della vescica urinaria | Rupture of urinary bladder |
| Rottura di aneurisma | Aneurysm rupture |
| Rottura muscolare | Muscle rupture |
| Ruga | Wrinkle |
| Rumore durante la respirazione (stridore) | Breathing sound due to blockage in the airway (stridor) |
| Sacco dell'ernia | Hernia sack |
| Salmonellosi | Salmonellosis |
| Sangue al liquido cerebrospinale | Blood in cerebrospinal fluid |
| Sangue nelle feci (ematochezia) | Blood in stool (hematochezia) |
| Sangue nello sputo (emottisi) | Blood in sputum (hemoptysis) |
| Sarcoidosi | Sarcoidosis (sarcoid, Besnier-Boeck disease) |
| Sarcoma | Sarcoma |
| Sarcoma botrioide | Botryoid sarcoma |
| Sarcoma di Ewing | Ewing's sarcoma |
| Sarcoma di Kaposi | Kaposi's sarcoma |
| Sarcoma sinoviale | Synovial sarcoma |
| Sarcopenia | Sarcopenia |
| SARS (Sindrome Acuta Respiratoria Severa) | Severe acute respiratory syndrome (SARS) |
| Sbadiglio | Yawn |
| Sbavando (ptialismo, scialorrea) | Drooling (ptyalism, sialorrhea, slobbering) |
| Scabbia (rogna) | Scabies (the itch) |
| Scarlattina | Scarlet fever |
| Scarsa secrezione salivare (xerostomia) | Dry mouth (xerostomia) |
| Schistosomiasi | Schistosomiasis (snail fever) |
| Schizofrenia | Schizophrenia |
| Sciatica | Sciatica |
| Sclerodermia | Scleroderma |
| Sclerosi laterale amiotrofica | Amyotrophic lateral sclerosis |
| Sclerosi multipla | Multiple sclerosis |
| Scoliosi | Scoliosis |
| Scorbuto | Scurvy |
| Scossa muscolare (fasciciolazione) | Muscle twitch (fasciculation) |
| Scotoma | Scotoma |
| Seborrea | Seborrhea |
| Semi-coma | Semicoma |
| Sensazione bruciante | Burning sensation |
| Sensibilità al dolore (algesia) | Sensitivity to pain (algesia) |
| Senso della paura | Sensation of fear |
| Senso delle scarpe troppo strette | 'Tight shoes' sensation |
| Sepsi | Sepsis |
| Sesta malattia (roseola infantum, esantema subitum) | Exanthema subitum (roseola infantum, sixth disease) |
| Sete | Thirst |
| Setticemia | Septicemia |
| Sfogo (eruzione cutanea) | Rash (eruption, eczema) |
| Shigellosi | Shigellosis (bacillary dysentery) |
| Shock cardiogeno | Cardiogenic shock |
| Shock chirurgico | Surgical shock (postoperative shock) |
| Shock endotossico | Endotoxic shock |
| Shock ipovolemico | Hypovolemic shock |
| Shock neurogeno | Neurogenic shock |
| Shock ostruttivo | Obstructive shock |
| Shock settico | Septic shock |
| Shock spinale | Spinal shock |
| Shock traumatico | Traumatic shock |
| SIDA (sindrome da ImmunoDeficienza Acquisita, AIDS) | AIDS (acquired immune deficiency syndrome) |
| Siderosi | Siderosis |
| Sifilide (lue) | Syphilis |
| Sifiloma | Chancre |
| Silicosi | Silicosis |
| Sincope | Syncope |
| Sindattilia | Syndactyly |
| Sindrome alcolica fetale | Fetal alcohol syndrome |
| Sindrome cervicale | Cervicocephal syndrome |
| Sindrome cervicobrachiale (sindrome spalla-mano) | Cervicobrachial syndrome |
| Sindrome compartimentale | Compartment syndrome |
| Sindrome da carcinoide | Carcinoid syndrome |
| Sindrome da conflitto subacromiale (impingement sub-acromiale) | Shoulder impingement syndrome (subacromial impingement syndrome) |
| Sindrome da distress respiratorio | Respiratory distress syndrome |

| | |
|---|---|
| Sindrome da distress respiratorio del neonato (malattia da membrane ialine polmonari) | Hyaline membrane disease (infant respiratory distress syndrome) |
| Sindrome da fatica cronica | Chronic fatigue syndrome |
| Sindrome da impingement della caviglia | Ankle impingement syndrome |
| Sindrome da impingement posteriore di caviglia | Posterior ankle impingement syndrome |
| Sindrome da schiacciamento | Crush-syndrome |
| Sindrome da stress tibiale mediale | Shin splints |
| Sindrome da vibrazioni mano-braccio | Hand-arm vibration syndrome (vibration white finger) |
| Sindrome degli ischio-crurali (sindrome dell'hamstring) | Tight hamstrings syndrome |
| Sindrome del bambino flaccido | Floppy infant syndrome |
| Sindrome del colon irritabile (colon spastico) | Irritable bowel syndrome (spastic colon) |
| Sindrome del dolore patello-femorale (ginocchio del corridore) | Chondromalacia patellae (runner's knee, patello-femoral pain syndrome) |
| Sindrome del grido di gatto | Cat cry syndrome (5p minus syndrome, Lejeune's syndrome) |
| Sindrome del tunnel carpale | Carpal tunnel syndrome |
| Sindrome del tunnel cubitale | Little league elbow syndrome (LLE syndrome) |
| Sindrome del tunnel tarsale | Tarsal tunnel syndrome |
| Sindrome della benderella ileotibiale | Iliotibial band friction syndrome |
| Sindrome della classe economica | Traveller's thrombosis (economy class syndrome) |
| Sindrome della morte improvvisa del lattante | Sudden infant death syndrome (crib death, cot death) |
| Sindrome delle apnee nel sonno | Sleep apnea |
| Sindrome dello stretto toracico superiore | Thoracic outlet syndrome |
| Sindrome di Behçet | Behçet's disease |
| Sindrome di Blount | Blount's disease |
| Sindrome di Cushing (ipercortisolismo) | Cushing's syndrome (hypercorticism) |
| Sindrome di De Quervain | DeQuervain syndrome |
| Sindrome di Down | Down syndrome |
| Sindrome di Edwards | Edwards syndrome (trisomy 18) |
| Sindrome di Eisenmenger | Eisenmenger's syndrome |
| Sindrome di Goodpasture | Goodpasture's syndrome |
| Sindrome di Guillain-Barré | Guillain-Barré syndrome |
| Sindrome di Hoffa | Hoffa's disease |
| Sindrome di Kawasaki | Kawasaki disease |
| Sindrome di Leriche | Aortoiliac occlusive disease (Leriche's syndrome) |
| Sindrome di Marfan | Marfan syndrome |
| Sindrome di McCune-Albright-Sternberg | McCune-Albright syndrome |
| Sindrome di Menière | Meniere's disease |
| Sindrome di Osgood-Schlatter | Osgood-Schlatter disease (rugby knee) |
| Sindrome di Patau | Patau syndrome (trisomy 13) |
| Sindrome di Preiser | Preiser disease |
| Sindrome di Raynaud | Raynaud's disease |
| Sindrome di Reiter | Reactive arthritis (Reiter's syndrome) |
| Sindrome di Reye | Reye's syndrome |
| Sindrome di Sjögren | Sjögren's syndrome |
| Sindrome di Tourette | Tourette's syndrome |
| Sindrome di Turner | Turner syndrome |
| Sindrome dolorosa | Pain syndrome |
| Sindrome epato-renale | Hepatorenal syndrome |
| Sindrome mielodisplasica | Myelodysplastic syndrome |
| Sindrome nefrosica | Nephrotic syndrome |
| Sindrome post trombotica | Post-thrombotic syndrome |
| Sindrome premestruale | Premenstrual syndrome (PMS) |
| Sindrome prodromica | Early symptom (prodrome) |
| Singhiozzo | Hiccup |
| Sinostosi radio-ulnare | Radioulnar synostosis |
| Sinovioma | Synovioma |
| Sinusite | Sinus headache |
| Siringomielia | Syringomyelia |
| Soffio cardiaco | Heart murmur |

| | |
|---|---|
| Soffocamento (soffocazione, asfissia) | Choking (suffocation) |
| Sonnambulismo | Sleepwalking (somnambulism) |
| Sonnolenza | Somnolence |
| Soppressione della secrezione di urina | Nonpassage of urine |
| Sordità | Deafness |
| Sordità parziale | Hard of hearing |
| Sottopeso (grave magrezza) | Underfedness (malnutrition) |
| Spasmo (contrazione involontaria) | Spasm (cramp) |
| Spasmo di vagina (vaginismo) | Vaginal spasm (vaginismus) |
| Spasmo facciale | Facial spasm |
| Spasmo muscolare | Muscular cramp (spasm) |
| Spermatocele (cisti spermatica) | Spermatocele |
| Spina bifida | Spina bifida |
| Spina nel calcagno (spina calcaneare) | Heel spur (calcaneal spur) |
| Splenomegalia | Splenomegaly |
| Spondilite | Spondylitis |
| Spondilite anchilosante | Ankylosing spondylitis (Bechterew's syndrome) |
| Spondilite tubercolare (morbo di Pott) | Tuberculous spondylitis (Pott disease) |
| Spondilolistesi | Spondylolisthesis |
| Spondilosi | Spondylosis |
| Sporotricosi | Sporotrichosis |
| Spostamento del rene (ptosi renale, nefroptosi) | Floating kidney (nephroptosis, renal ptosis) |
| Spostamento della palpebra (palpebra calante, blefaroptosi) | Drooping of the upper eyelid (blepharoptosis) |
| Sputo schiumoso | Foamy sputum |
| Stanchezza (fatica, astenia) | Fatigue (exhaustion, lethargy) |
| Starnuto | Sneezing |
| Stenosi aortica | Aortic valve stenosis |
| Stenosi dell'arteria polmonare | Stenosis of pulmonary artery |
| Stenosi esofagea | Esophageal stenosis |
| Stenosi ipertrofica del piloro | Hypertrophic pyloric stenosis |
| Stenosi mitralica | Mitral stenosis |
| Stenosi pilorica | Pyloric stenosis |
| Stenosi pilorica congenita | Congenital pyloric stenosis |
| Stenosi polmonare | Pulmonary valve stenosis |
| Sterilità (infecondità) | Infertility (sterility) |
| Stiramento | Strain (sprain, pull) |
| Stiramento del legamento | Ligament sprain |
| Stiramento del tendine | Tendon strain |
| Stitichezza (costipazione) | Constipation (obstipation) |
| Strabismo | Strabismus |
| Strangolamento (strozzamento) | Strangulation |
| Strappo muscolare | Muscle strain (muscle pull) |
| Stupor | Sopor |
| Stupore | Stupor |
| Sudorazione (traspirazione) | Sweating |
| Sudore notturno | Night sweats |
| Tachicardia | Tachycardia |
| Talassemia | Thalassemia |
| Tamponamento cardiaco | Pericardial tamponade (cardiac tamponade) |
| Tappo di cerume | Impacted cerumen |
| Temperatura corporea elevata | Elevated body temperature |
| Tendinite dei estensori delle dita del piede | Extensor tendinitis (inflammation of the extensor tendons of the toes) |
| Tendinite del flessore lungo dell'alluce | Dancer's tendinitis (flexor hallucis tendinitis) |
| Tendinite del muscolo tibiale posteriore | Tibialis posterior tendinitis |
| Tendinite del popliteo | Popliteus syndrome |
| Tendinite dell'avambraccio | Forearm tendinitis |
| Tendinopatia Achille da overuse | Achilles tendon overuse injury |
| Tendinopatia achillea (achillodinia) | Achillodynia (Achilles tendinitis) |
| Tendinosi | Tendinosis (chronic tendon injury) |
| Tensione di parete addominale | Abdominal wall tension |
| Teratocarcinoma | Teratocarcinoma |
| Teratoma | Teratoma |
| Tetania | Tetany |
| Tetano | Tetanus |
| Tetralogia di Fallot | Tetralogy of Fallot |
| Tic | Tic |
| Tifo esantematico (tifo epidemico) | Epidemic typhus (louse-borne typhus) |
| Tifo murino (tifo endemico) | Murine typhus (endemic typhus) |
| Tigna (tinea capitis) | Tinea capitis (scalp ringworm) |
| Tinea corporis | Tinea corporis |

| | |
|---|---|
| Tinea cruris | Crotch itch (tinea cruris) |
| Tinea favosa | Favus |
| Tirare su col naso | Sniffing (sniffle) |
| Tireotossicosi | Thyrotoxicosis |
| Tiroidite di Hashimoto | Hashimoto's disease |
| Tiroidite di Riedel | Riedel's thyroiditis |
| Torace a imbuto (petto escavato) | Pectus excavatum |
| Torcicollo | Wry neck (torticollis) |
| Torsione del testicolo | Testicular torsion |
| Torsione dell'osso | Bone bending (bone torsion) |
| Tosse | Cough |
| Tosse produttiva | Productive cough |
| Tosse secca | Dry cough |
| Tossicodipendenza (tossicomania) | Drug addiction |
| Tossinfezione da Clostridium perfringens | Clostridium perfringens toxic infection |
| Toxocariasi | Toxocariasis |
| Toxoplasmosi | Toxoplasmosis |
| Tracoma | Trachoma |
| Trapianto renale | Kidney transplatation |
| Trasposizione dei grossi vasi | Transposition of the great vessels |
| Trasposizione dell'aorta | Transposition of aorta |
| Trasposizione dell'arteria polmonare | Transposition of pulmonary artery |
| Trauma sportivo | Sports injury |
| Tremito (tremore) | Tremor |
| Tremore delle mani | Hand tremor |
| Trichinosi | Trichinosis (trichinellosis) |
| Trichomonas vaginalis | Trichomonas vaginalis |
| Trichomoniasi | Trichomoniasis |
| Tripanosomiasi | Trypanosomiasis |
| Tripanosomiasi africana (malattia del sonno) | African trypanosomiasis (sleeping sickness) |
| Trombo | Blood clot (thrombus) |
| Trombocitopenia | Thrombocytopenia |
| Tromboembolia | Thromboembolism |
| Tromboflebite | Thrombophlebitis |
| Trombosi | Thrombosis |
| Trombosi venosa | Venous thrombosis |
| Tsutsugamushi (tifo fluviale giapponese) | Scrub typhus (Japanese river fever, Tsutsugamushi fever) |
| Tubercolosi (tisi) | Tuberculosis (TBC) |
| Tubercolosi dei reni | Renal tuberculosis |
| Tubercolosi delle ossa | Bone tuberculosis |
| Tubercolosi epatica | Hepatic tuberculosis |
| Tubercolosi intestinale | Intestinal tuberculosis |
| Tubercolosi polmonare | Pulmonary tuberculosis |
| Tubercolosi urogenitale | Urogenital tuberculosis |
| Tularemia (febbre dei conigli) | Tularemia (rabbit fever) |
| Tumore | Tumor (tumour) |
| Tumore benigno | Benign tumor |
| Tumore del sacco vitellino | Yolk sac tumor (endodermal sinus tumor) |
| Tumore di Brenner | Brenner tumour |
| Tumore di Wilms (nefroblastoma) | Wilm's tumor (nephroblastoma) |
| Tumore maligno | Malignant tumor (cancer) |
| Tumore misto | Mixed tumor |
| Tumore misto maligno | Malignant mixed tumor |
| Tungiasi (tunga penetrans) | Tungiasis (nigua, pique) |
| Ulcera (ulcerazione) | Ulcer |
| Ulcera duodenale | Duodenal ulcer |
| Ulcera gastrica | Gastric ulcer |
| Ulcera ischemica | Ischemic ulceration |
| Ulcera perforata | Perforated ulcer |
| Ulcera varicosa | Venous ulcer (varicose ulcer) |
| Ulcera venerea (cancroide) | Chancroid (soft chancre) |
| Unghia incarnita (onicocriptosi) | Ingrown nail (onychocryptosis, unguis incarnatus) |
| Uremia (accumulo nel sangue di sostanze azotate a causa dell'insufficienza renale) | Uremia (autointoxication due to kidney failure) |
| Urina di colore rosso | Red urine |
| Urina marrone | Brown urine |
| Urinazione frequente (pollachiuria) | Frequent urination |
| Urinazione notturna (nicturia) | Frequent urination at night (nocturia) |
| Urine torbide | Unclear urine (foggy urine) |
| Ustione | Burn |
| Ustione da corrente elettrica | Electric shock burn |
| Ustione da medusa | Jellyfish sting burn |
| Vampata di calore | Hot flushes |
| Varicella | Chicken-pox |
| Varici degli arti inferiori | Leg varicose veins |

| | |
|---|---|
| Varici esofagee | Esophageal varices |
| Varicocele | Varicocele |
| Varicosi (varici, malattia varicosa) | Varicose veins |
| Variola vera (vaiolo) | Smallpox |
| Vene varicose del collo | Neck varicose veins |
| Verruca | Wart |
| Vescichetta (bolla) | Blister |
| Visione doppia (diplopia) | Double vision (diplopia) |
| Vitiligine | Vitiligo |
| Voglia (neo, nevo) | Birthmark (nevus) |
| Volvolo | Abnormal twisting of the intestines (volvulus) |
| Vomito (emetismo) | Vomiting |
| Vomito senza nausea (vomito a getto, vomito cerebrale) | Vomiting without nausea (cerebral vomiting) |
| Xantelasma | Xanthelasma |
| Xantoma | Xanthoma |
| Zoonosi | Zoonosis |
| Zoppicamento | Limping |

## FARMACIA — PHARMACY

| | |
|---|---|
| A digiuno | On an empty stomach (before the meal) |
| A mezzogiorno | At noon |
| Acido borico | Boric acid |
| Adrenalina | Adrenaline |
| Aerosol | Aerosol |
| Ago | Needle |
| Alcool | Alcohol |
| Allergia a medicamento | Drug allergy |
| Aminofillina | Aminophylline |
| Ampicillina | Ampicillin |
| Ampolla (fiala) | Ampoule |
| Analgesico | Analgesic (painkiller) |
| Anestetico | Anesthetic |
| Antiacido | Antacid |
| Antibiotico | Antibiotic |
| Anticoagulante | Anticoagulant |
| Anticonvulsante | Anticonvulsant |
| Antidepressivo | Antidepressant |
| Antidiabetico | Anti-diabetic drug |
| Antidiaforetico | Antiperspirant |
| Antidiarroici | Antidiarrhoeal drug |
| Antidoto | Antidote |
| Antielmintici | Antihelminthic |
| Antiemetico | Antiemetic and motion sickness drug |
| Antimalarico | Antimalarial drug |
| Antimicotico | Antimycotic |
| Antinfiammatorio | Anti-inflammatory |
| Antiossidante (sostanza antiossidante) | Antioxidant |
| Antipiretico | Antipyretic |
| Antipsicotico | Antipsychotic |
| Antireumatico | Antirheumatic drug |
| Antisettico | Antiseptic |
| Antisettico urinario | Urinary antiseptic |
| Antisiero | Antiserum |
| Antistaminico | Antihistamine |
| Antitossina | Antitoxin |
| Aspirina | Aspirin |
| Assorbenti igienici | Sanitary pads (sanitary napkins) |
| Assorbenti per l'incontinenza | Incontinence pads (adult diapers) |
| Atropina | Atropine |
| Barbiturico | Barbiturate |
| Bendaggio | Bandage |
| Bilancia | Scales |
| Bottiglietta (boccetta) | Vial |
| Bouillotte (bouilloire) | Hot water bottle |
| Broncodilatatore | Bronchodilator |
| Burrocacao | Lip balm |
| Caffeina | Caffeine |
| Calcio | Calcium |
| Camomilla | Chamomile |
| Candelette | Vaginal suppository |
| Cannabis terapeutica | Medical cannabis |
| Capsula | Capsule |
| Carbone attivo | Activated carbon |
| Cardiotonico | Cardiotonic agent |
| Cefalosporina | Cephalosporin |
| Cerotto | Plaster (adhesive strip) |
| Cerotto antifumo | Nicotine patch |
| Chemioterapia | Chemotherapy |
| Citostatico | Cytostatic |
| Clistere | Enema (clyster) |
| Cloramfenicolo | Chloramphenicol |
| Cloro | Chlorine |
| Cobalto | Cobalt |
| Codeina | Codeine |
| Collirio | Eye drops |
| Collutorio | Mouthwash liquid |
| Compressa | Compress |
| Compressa (pasticca, tavoletta) | Tablet |
| Compresse solubili | Water-soluble tablets |
| Contraccettivo | Contraceptive |
| Corticosteroide | Corticosteroid |
| Crema | Skin cream |
| Cucchiaio | Spoon |
| Dentifricio | Tooth paste |
| Di mattina | In the morning |
| Diaframma | Diaphragm (Dutch cap) |
| Digestivo | Digestive |

| | |
|---|---|
| Dimagrante (farmaco antiobesità) | Anti-obesity medication |
| Diuretico | Diuretic |
| Dolcificante artificiale | Sugar substitute |
| Dopo il pasto | After meal |
| Dose | Dose |
| Effetti indesiderati da farmaco | Drug side-effects |
| Emostatico | Antihemorrhagic (hemostatic) |
| Emulsione | Emulsion |
| Eparina | Heparin |
| Eritromicina | Erythromycin |
| Espettorante | Expectorant |
| Farmacista | Pharmacist |
| Farmaco anti-alcol | Antialcoholic drug |
| Farmaco antiinfiammatore non steroide FANS | Non-steroidal anti-inflammatory drug |
| Farmaco antiallergico | Antiallergic drug |
| Farmaco antianemico | Antianemic |
| Farmaco antiaritmico | Antiarrhythmic agent |
| Farmaco antiipertensivo | Antihypertensive drug |
| Farmaco antiprotozoico | Antiprotozoal agent |
| Farmaco antitubercolare | Antitubercular agent |
| Farmaco antivirale | Antiviral drug |
| Fentanyl | Fentanyl |
| Ferro | Iron |
| Filo interdentale | Dental floss |
| Filtro solare (crema solare ad alta protezione) | Sunscreen (sunblock) |
| Fitoterapia | Phytotherapy |
| Fosforo | Phosphorus |
| Garza | Gauze sponge |
| Gel | Gel |
| Gentamicina | Gentamicin |
| Glucosio | Glucose |
| Gocce | Drops |
| Gocce nasali | Nasal drops |
| Gocce per il mal di orecchi | Ear drops |
| Gomma da masticare antifumo | Nicotine gum |
| Grammo | Gram (gramme) |
| Immunoglobulina | Immunoglobulin |
| Immunosoppressivo | Immunosuppressive |
| Inalazione (farmaco per inalazioni) | Inhalation |
| Iniezione | Injection |
| Insettifugo | Insect repellent |
| Insulina | Insulin |
| Interferone | Interferon |
| Iodio (tintura di iodio) | Iodine |
| Ipnotico | Hypnotic (soporific) |
| La sera | In the evening |
| Lassativo | Laxative |
| Lente a contatto morbida | Soft contact lens |
| Lente a contatto rigida | Hard contact lens |
| Lenti a contatto | Contact lenses |
| Litro | Litre |
| Lozione | Lotion |
| Lubrificante | Lubricant |
| Magnesio | Magnesium |
| Manganese | Manganese |
| Medicamento (farmaco, rimedio) | Medication (remedy, drug) |
| Metadone | Methadone |
| Microgrammo | Microgram |
| Milligrammo | Milligram (milligramme) |
| Millilitro | Millilitre |
| Minerale | Mineral |
| Miorilassante | Muscle relaxant |
| Misuratore di pressione (sfigmomanometro) | Blood pressure meter (sphygmomanometer) |
| Molibdeno | Molybdenum |
| Morfina | Morphine |
| Mucolitico | Mucolytic |
| Nistatina | Nystatin |
| Occhiali | Glasses |
| Olio di jojoba | Jojoba oil |
| Olio di mandorla | Almond oil |
| Olio di ricino | Castor oil |
| Olio essenziale (olio eterico) | Essential oil |
| Olio minerale | Mineral oil |
| Omega-3 acidi grassi | Omega-3 fatty acid |
| Oppioide | Opioid |
| Oralmente (per via orale, per bocca) | Orally |
| Ossicodone | Oxycodone |
| Ovatta | Cotton-wool |
| Paracetamolo | Paracetamol |
| Paraffina | Paraffin |
| Pezzo (porzione) | Piece |
| Pasta | Paste |
| Pasticca (pastiglia) | Pastille (lozenge) |
| Penicillina | Penicillin |
| Per l'applicazione esterna | For external application |
| Pillola anticoncezionale | Contraceptive pill (oral contraceptive) |
| Pillola del "giorno doppo" (contraccezione postcoitale, contraccezione di emergenza) | 'Morning-after' pill (postcoital contraception, emergency contraception) |
| Polvere liquido | Liquid powder |

| | |
|---|---|
| Polverina (polvere) | Powder |
| Pomata (unguento) | Ointment (fat) |
| Potassio | Potassium |
| Pozione | Potion |
| Prescrizione (rimedio prescritto) | Prescription |
| Preservativo (profilattico, condom) | Condom |
| Psicostimulanti | Psychostimulant |
| Purgante (purga) | Purgative |
| Rame | Copper |
| Repellente antizanzare | Mosquito repellent |
| Rettale | Rectal |
| Salicilato | Salicylate |
| Sapone | Soap |
| Schiuma (spuma) | Foam |
| Schiuma anticoncezionale | Contraceptive foam |
| Sciacquatra (risciacquatura) | Rinsing |
| Sciroppo | Syrup |
| Sedativo (calmante) | Sedative |
| Siero | Serum |
| Siringa per iniezioni | Syringe |
| Sistema internazionale di unità di misura | International System of Units |
| Sodio | Sodium |
| Soluzione | Solution |
| Soluzione fisiologica | Saline solution |
| Soluzione per pulizia dentiera | Denture cleaning solution |
| Soluzione per pulizia lenti a contatto | Contact lenses cleaning solution |
| Sostanza nutriente (sostanza nutritiva) | Nutrient |
| Sovradosaggio | Overdose |
| Spasmolitico | Spasmolytic |
| Spermicida | Spermicide |
| Spruzzo (vaporizzato) | Spray |
| Spugna contraccettiva | Contraceptive sponge |
| Sublinguale | Sublingual administration |
| Sulfamidici (sulfonamidici) | Sulphonamide |
| Supposta | Suppository |
| Tampone | Tampon |
| Terapia ormonale sostitutiva | Hormone replacement therapy |
| Termometro | Thermometer |
| Test di gravidanza ad uso domiciliare | Home pregnancy test |
| Tetraciclina | Tetracycline |
| Tintura | Tincture |
| Tisana (infuso di erbe) | Herbal tea |
| Tonico (ricostituente) | Tonic |
| Tramadolo | Tramadol |
| Vaccino | Vaccine |
| Vasodilatatore | Vasodilatator |
| Veleno | Poison |
| Viagra (citrato di sildenafil) | Viagra (sildenafil citrate) |
| Vitamina | Vitamin |
| Vitamina A (retinolo) | Vitamin A (retinol) |
| Vitamina B1 (tiamina) | Vitamin B1 (thiamin) |
| Vitamina B2 (riboflavina) | Vitamin B2 (riboflavin) |
| Vitamina B3 (niacina, vitamina PP) | Vitamin B3 (niacin) |
| Vitamina B4 (adenina) | Vitamin B4 (adenine) |
| Vitamina B5 (acido pantotenico, vitamina W) | Vitamin B5 (pantothenic acid) |
| Vitamina B6 (piridossina) | Vitamin B6 (pyridoxine) |
| Vitamina B7 (inositolo) | Vitamin B7 (inositol) |
| Vitamina B8 (biotina) | Vitamin B8 (biotin) |
| Vitamina B9 (acido folico) | Vitamin B9 (folic acid) |
| Vitamina B10 (vitamina R) | Vitamin B10 (factor-R) |
| Vitamina B11 (vitamina S) | Vitamin B11 (factor-S) |
| Vitamina B12 (cobalamina) | Vitamin B12 (cobalamin) |
| Vitamina C (acido L-ascorbico) | Vitamin C (L-ascorbic acid) |
| Vitamina D2 (ergocalciferolo) | Vitamin D2 (ergocalciferol) |
| Vitamina D3 (colecalciferolo) | Vitamin D3 (cholecalciferol) |
| Vitamina D4 (diidro-ergocalciferolo) | Vitamin D4 |
| Vitamina D5 (sitocalciferolo) | Vitamin D5 (sitocalciferol) |
| Vitamina E (tocoferolo) | Vitamin E (tocopherol) |
| Vitamina F (acido linoleico) | Vitamin F (linoleic acid) |
| Vitamina J (colina) | Vitamin J (choline) |
| Vitamina K (fillochinone) | Vitamin K (phylloquinone) |
| Vitamina L1 (acido antranilico) | Vitamin L1 (anthranilic acid) |
| Vitamina P (flavonoidi) | Vitamin P (flavonoids) |
| Zinco | Zinc |
| Zinco pasta | Zinc ointment |
| Zolfo | Sulphur |

| ISTITUZIONI, PROCEDURE E CURE DI MEDICINA | MEDICAL FACILITIES, PROCEDURES AND CARE |
|---|---|
| Accettazione | Reception office |
| Acqua | Water |
| Addentare | Bite |
| Allarme | Alarm |
| Ambulanza | Ambulance (clinic) |
| Amputazione | Amputation |
| Anestesia | Anesthesia |
| Anestesia generale | General anesthesia |
| Anestesia locale | Local anesthesia |
| Angioplastica coronarica | Percutaneous coronary intervention (coronary angioplasty) |
| Apertura chirurgica del cranio (craniotomia) | Surgical opnening of the cranium (craniotomy) |
| Apertura chirurgica di un articolazione (artrotomia) | Surgical procedure on a joint (arthrotomy) |
| Apparecchio acustico | Hearing assist device |
| Aprire | Open |
| Armadio (credenza) | Wardrobe (cupboard, cabinet) |
| Artrodesi | Arthrodesis |
| Ascensore | Elevator |
| Aspiratore di secreti | Suction unit (aspirator) |
| Asportazione chirurgica del pancreas (pancreatectomia) | Surgical removal of the pancreas (pancreatectomy) |
| Asportazione chirurgica del testicolo (orchiectomia) | Surgical removal of a testicle (orchidectomy) |
| Asportazione chirurgica del timo (timectomia) | Surgical removal of the thymus (thymectomy) |
| Asportazione chirurgica dell'appendice (appendicectomia) | Surgical removal of the vermiform appendix (appendectomy) |
| Asportazione chirurgica dell'utero (isterectomia) | Surgical removal of the uterus (hysterectomy) |
| Asportazione chirurgica della colecisti (colecistectomia) | Surgical removal of the gallbladder (cholecystectomy) |
| Asportazione chirurgica della lamina di vertebre (laminectomia) | Surgical procedure on the spine (laminectomy) |
| Asportazione chirurgica della laringe (laringectomia) | Surgical removal of the larynx (laryngectomy) |
| Asportazione chirurgica della mammella (mastectomia) | Surgical removal of a breast (mastectomy) |
| Asportazione chirurgica della milza (splenectomia) | Surgical removal of the spleen (splenectomy) |
| Asportazione chirurgica della prostata (prostatectomia) | Surgical removal of the prostate gland (prostatectomy) |
| Asportazione chirurgica della sacca aneurismatica (aneurismectomia) | Surgical removal of the aneurysm (aneurysmectomy) |
| Asportazione chirurgica della tiroide (tiroidectomia) | Surgical removal of the thyroid gland (thyroidectomy) |
| Asportazione chirurgica delle adenoidi (adenoidectomia) | Surgical removal of adenoids (adenoidectomy) |
| Asportazione chirurgica delle emorroidi (emorroidectomia) | Surgical removal of a hemorrhoid (hemorrhoidectomy) |
| Asportazione chirurgica delle tonsille (tonsillectomia) | Surgical removal of tonsils (tonsillectomy) |
| Asportazione chirurgica dello stomaco (gastrectomia) | Surgical removal of the stomach (gastrectomy) |
| Asportazione chirurgica di calcolo (litotomia) | Surgical removal of stones (lithotomy) |
| Asportazione chirurgica di fibromi nell'utero (miomectomia) | Surgical removal of uterine myomas (myomectomy, fibroidectomy) |
| Asportazione chirurgica di strutturalobale di un organo (lobectomia) | Surgical removal of a lobe of some organ (lobectomy) |
| Asportazione chirurgica di uno o etrambi surreni (surrenectomia, adrenalectomia) | Surgical removal of one or both adrenal glands (adrenalectomy) |
| Assicurazione sanitaria | Health insurance |
| Assistenza infermieristica | Nursing (care) |

| | |
|---|---|
| Assistenza sanitaria primaria | Primary health care |
| Autoambulanza | Ambulance |
| Autopsia | Autopsy |
| Bagno | Bathroom |
| Barella (lettiga) | Stretcher |
| Bendaggio gessato | Plaster cast (immobilization plaster) |
| Bypass | Bypass |
| Cadavere (salma) | Corpse |
| Calendario vaccinale | Vaccination schedule |
| Cambiarsi | Get changed |
| Camera di malato | Patient's room |
| Camicia da notte | Nightgown |
| Camicia protettiva | Protection gown |
| Cannula | Airway (cannula) |
| Cannula nasale | Nasal cannula |
| Cannula oro-faringea | Oropharyngeal airway |
| Cardiologia | Cardiology |
| Cardiostimolatore (stimolatore cardiaco) | Pacemaker |
| Carrello | Hospital trolley |
| Carrell servitore | Overbed table |
| Cassetta di pronto soccorso | First aid kit |
| Catetere | Catheter |
| Catetere vescicale | Urological catheter |
| Causa di morte | Cause of death |
| Cauterizzazione | Cauterization |
| Cena | Dinner (supper) |
| Centro di medicina | Medical center |
| Chemioterapia | Chemotherapy |
| Chirurgia | Surgery |
| Chirurgia laparoscopica | Laparoscopic surgery |
| Chiudere | Close |
| Chiusura delle tube | Surgical sterilization of a woman (tubal ligation) |
| Ciabatte | Slippers |
| Circoncisione | Circumcision |
| Citologia | Cytology |
| Colazione | Breakfast |
| Collare cervicale | Neck immobilizer |
| Comodino | Night table (bedside table) |
| Contagioso (infettivo) | Contagious |
| Coperta | Cover |
| Corona | Dental crown |
| Crioestrazione | Cryoextraction |
| Cuffietta protettiva | Protection cap |
| Cuscino | Pillow |
| Deambulatore (tutore per disabili) | Walker (walking frame) |
| Defecazione | Defecation |
| Defibrillatore | Defibrillator |
| Defibrillatore manuale | Manual defibrillator |
| Defibrillazione | Defibrillation |
| Dentista | Dentist |
| Deposito (magazzino) | Storage |
| Dermatologia | Dermatology |
| Diagnosi | Diagnosis |
| Dialisi | Dialysis |
| Dialisi epatica | Liver dialysis |
| Dialisi renale | Renal dialysis |
| Dieta (regime dietetico) | Diet |
| Digestione | Digestion |
| Dinamometro | Dynamometer |
| Donatore / donatrice | Donor |
| Donazione del sangue | Blood donation |
| Dottore / dottoressa (medico) | Doctor (physician) |
| Drenaggio | Drainage |
| Drenaggio posturale | Postural drainage |
| Elettrochirurgia | Electrosurgery |
| Elettrodo | Electrode |
| Elettroterapia | Electrotherapy |
| Esercizi di equilibrio | Balance training |
| Esercizi di Kegel | Kegel exercise |
| Esercizi di respirazione | Breathing exercises |
| Esercizio | Exercise |
| Estrazione del dente | Dental extraction |
| Fasciatura (bendaggio) | Dressing |
| Fermacapo | Head immobilizer |
| Finestra | Window |
| Fisioterapia | Physical therapy |
| Fisioterapista | Physiotherapist |
| Forbici | Scissors |
| Formazione chirurgica di stomia (colostomia) | Surgical procedure of formation of stoma (colostomy) |
| Gel elettro-conduttivo | Electrode conductive gel |
| Germi | Germs |
| Gerontologia | Gerontology |
| Ginecologia | Gynecology |
| Goniometro | Goniometer |
| Gruccia (stampella) | Crutch |
| Guanti protettivi | Protect gloves |
| Guarigione (ristabilimento) | Recovery |
| Idroterapia | Hydrotherapy |
| Immunologia | Immunology |
| Incisione chirurgica della trachea (tracheotomia) | Surgical opening of a direct airway on the neck (tracheostomy) |
| Infermiera /infermiere | Nurse |
| Infusione | Infusion |

| | |
|---|---|
| Iniezione | Injection |
| Intervento chirurgico dell'orecchio medio (stapedectomia) | Surgical procedure on the middle ear (stapedectomy) |
| Intervento chirurgico delle connessioni talamiche (talamotomia) | Surgical procedure on the thalamus (thalamotomy) |
| Intubazione | Intubation |
| Laringoscopio | Laryngoscope |
| Lavanda gastrica | Gastric lavage (stomach pumping) |
| Lavanderia | Laundry |
| Lavare (fare il bagno) | Bath (wash) |
| Lenzuolo | Sheet |
| Letto | Bed |
| Lift facciale (ritidectomia) | Facelift (rhytidectomy) |
| Liposuzione | Liposuction |
| Lobotomia | Lobotomy |
| Luce | Light |
| Manicotto di sfigmomanometro | Manometer cuff |
| Manovra di Heimlich | Heimlich maneuver (abdominal thrusts) |
| Maschera dell'ossigeno | Oxygen mask |
| Maschera laringea | Laryngeal mask airway |
| Maschera per rianimazione | CPR mask |
| Mascherina di protezione | Protection face mask |
| Materassino a depressione | Vacuum mattress |
| Materasso | Mattress |
| Medicina interna | Internal medicine |
| Medico di medicina generale (medico di famiglia) | General practitioner |
| Monitor per parametri vitali | Vital signs monitor |
| Morire | Die |
| Neurologia | Neurology |
| Obitorio (mortorio) | Morgue (mortuary) |
| Oncologia | Oncology |
| Operazione (intervento chirurgico) | Operation (surgery) |
| Ortopedia | Orthopedics |
| Ospedale (policlinico) | Hospital |
| Ospite (visitatore / visitatrice) | Visitor |
| Otorinolaringoiatria | Otorhinolaryngology |
| Otturazione odontoiatrica | Dental filling |
| Padiglione (reparto) | Ward |
| Pallone autoespandibile | Ambu bag valve mask |
| Palpazione | Palpation |
| Patologia | Pathology |
| Pattumiera | Litter bin |
| Paziente (ammalato) | Patient |
| Pediatria | Pediatrics |
| Percussione | Percussion |
| Pessario | Pessary |
| Piantana portaflebo | Infusion stand |
| Pigiama | Pyjamas (pajamas) |
| Pinzette | Tweezers |
| Porta | Door |
| Posizionatore | Body positioner |
| Posizione di Trendelenburg | Trendelenburg position |
| Pranzo | Lunch |
| Primo soccorso | First aid |
| Procedura di chirurgia plastica del naso (rinoplastica) | Plastic surgery of the nose (rhinoplasty) |
| Procedura di chirurgia plastica del seno (mastoplastica) | Plastic surgery of the breasts (mammoplasty) |
| Procedura di chirurgia plastica dell'addome (addominoplastica) | Plastic surgery of the abdomen ("tummy tuck", abdominoplasty) |
| Procedura di chirurgia plastica della palpebra (blefaroplastica) | Plastic surgery of the eyelid (blepharoplasty) |
| Proclamazione del tempo della morte | Calling of the time of death |
| Proteggi materasso cerato | Incontinence pad |
| Protese mammaria | Breast implant |
| Protesi dentale | Dentures |
| Provetta | Test tube |
| Psichiatria | Psychiatry |
| Psicologo | Psychologist |
| Pulitura dei denti | Teeth polishing |
| Purificazione | Cleansing |
| Quarantena | Quarantine |
| Radiazione | Radiation |
| Radiologia | Radiology |
| Remissione | Remission |
| Reparto di malattie infettive | Infectious disease unit |
| Reparto di oftalmologia | Ophtalmology ward |
| Reparto polmonare | Pulmonary ward |
| Resezione transuretrale della prostata | Transurethral resection of the prostate |
| Respiratore | Respirator |
| Respirazione artificiale | Artificial respiration |

| | |
|---|---|
| Riabilitazione | Rehabilitation (rehab) |
| Rianimazione | Reanimation |
| Ricevente di trapianto | Recipient of an organ |
| Rinologia | Rhinology |
| Riposo a letto | Bed rest |
| Rottami | Debris |
| Sala d'aspetto | Waiting-room |
| Sala da pranzo (cenàcolo) | Dining-room |
| Sala operatoria | Operating room |
| Sanare (guarire, recuperare) | Recover (heal) |
| Scalpello | Scalpel |
| Sciacquare | Rinse |
| Secchia | Wash basin |
| Schiavina | Blanket |
| Sedia a rotelle (carrozzella) | Wheelchair |
| Sedia portantina | Escape chair |
| Serbatoio di ossigeno | Oxygen storage tank |
| Servizio di urgenza ed emergenza medica | Emergency medical services |
| Shunt | Shunt |
| Somministrazione dei farmaci | Administration of drugs |
| Sonda | Sonde |
| Sonda gastrica per nutrizione | Feeding tube |
| Sovrascarpe protettive | Protection shoe cover |
| Spugna | Sponge |
| Sputare | Spit |
| Stanza da terapia intensiva | Intensive care unit |
| Sterile | Sterile (aseptic) |
| Sterilizzazione | Sterilization |
| Stetofon endoscopio | Stethoscop |
| Suturare la ferita | Wound stitching |
| Talloniere e gomitiere antidecubito | Heel and elbow protectors |
| Tavolo (scrivania) | Table (desk) |
| Tè | Tea |
| Terapia | Therapy |
| Terapiaintensiva | Intensive care |
| Terapia semi-intensiva | Semi-intensive care |
| Terapista occupazionale | Occupational therapist |
| Trapano (trivella) | Drill |
| Trapianto | Transplantation |
| Trasfusione | Transfusion |
| Trauma | Trauma |
| Trazione | Traction |
| Tubo d'aspirazione | Suction catheter |
| Tubo di drenaggio | Drain tube |
| Tubo endotracheale | Endotracheal tube |
| Ufficio del medico | Doctor's office |
| Urinazione | Urination (voiding) |
| Urologia | Urology |
| Uso del gabinetto | Using a toilet |
| Vaccinazione (inoculazione) | Vaccination (inoculation) |
| Vasectomia | Surgical sterilization of a man (vasectomy) |
| Vaso da notte (pitale) | Chamber-pot |
| Vaso sanitario | Toilet (lavatory) |
| Visita | Visit |

## ESAMI MEDICI — MEDICAL EXAMS

| | |
|---|---|
| Agoaspirato (biopsia mediante ago sottile) | Fine needle aspiration biopsy |
| Agoaspirato polmonare percutaneo transtoracico | Transthoracic percutaneous fine needle aspiration |
| Amniocentesi | Amniocentesis |
| Analisi chimiche delle urine | Urine chemical analysis |
| Analisi dei gas nel sangue (emogas analisi) | Blood gas test |
| Analisi del DNA | DNA analysis |
| Analisi del liquido cerebro-spinale | Cerebrospinal fluid analysis |
| Angiografia | Angiography |
| Angiografia cerebrale | Cerebral angiography |
| Angiografia con cateterismo | Catheter angiography |
| Angiografia digitale a sottrazione | Digital subtraction angiography |
| Angiografia polmonare | Pulmonary angiography |
| Angiografia spinale | Spinal angiography |
| Anoscopia | Anoscopy |
| Antibiogramma | Antibiogram |
| Antigene carcino-embrionario (CEA) | Carcinoembryonic antigen (CEA) |
| Aortografia | Aortography |
| Arteriografia | Arteriography |
| Artrografia | Joint X-ray (arthrography) |
| Artroscopia | Arthroscopy |
| Aspartato transaminasi (SGOT) | Aspartate transaminase (SGOT) |
| Audiometria | Audiometry |
| Audiometria di discorso | Speech audiometry |
| Azoto ureico nel sangue (BUN) | Blood urea nitrogen test (BUN) |
| Biligrafia venosa | Intravenous biligraphy |
| Biomarcatore | Biomarker |

| | |
|---|---|
| Biopsia | Biopsy |
| Biopsia cerebrale (biopsia dei ventricoli cerebrali) | Brain ventricle biopsy |
| Biopsia cutanea | Skin biopsy |
| Biopsia del linfonodo | Lymph node biopsy |
| Biopsia del midollo osseo | Bone marrow biopsy |
| Biopsia della tiroide | Thyroid biopsy |
| Biopsia endometriale | Endometrial biopsy |
| Biopsia epatica | Liver biopsy |
| Biopsia pleurica | Pleural biopsy |
| Biopsia renale | Kidney biopsy |
| Biopsia stereotassica | Stereotactic biopsy |
| Broncografia | Bronchography |
| Broncoscopia | Bronchoscopy |
| CA 125 (antigene di carcinoma 125) | CA 125 (cancer antigen 125) |
| CA 19-9 (antigene carboidratico) | CA 19-9 (carbohydrate antigen) |
| Cardiotocografia | Cardiotocography |
| Cariotipo | Karyotype |
| Cateterismo cardiaco (angiocardiografia) | Cardiac catheterization (heart cath, angiocardiography) |
| Cefalometria | Cephalometry |
| Cistografia | Cystography |
| Cistoscopia | Cystoscopy |
| Colangio-pancreatografia endoscopica retrograda | Endoscopic retrograde cholangio-pancreatography (ERCP) |
| Colangiografia | Cholangiography |
| Colecistografia orale | Oral cholecystography |
| Colonscopia | Colonoscopy |
| Colposcopia | Colposcopy |
| Coltura del liquor | Cerebrospinal fluid culture |
| Coltura di gola | Throat swab culture |
| Coltura di microrganismi | Microbiological culture |
| Coltura di sputo | Sputum culture |
| Coltura vaginale | Vaginal swab culture |
| Concentrazione del glucosio nel plasma | Blood sugar concetration (glucose level) |
| Conizzazione | Cervical conization |
| Coronarografia | Coronary catheterization (coronarography) |
| Craniografia | Skull X-ray (craniography) |
| Defecografia | Defecography |
| Densità minerale ossea | Bone densitometry (dual energy X-ray absorpriometry) |
| Dermatoscopia (dermoscopia) | Dermatoscopy (dermoscopy) |
| Diagnosi differenziale | Differential diagnosis |
| Dilatazione delle pupille provocando con tropicamide | Drug induced pupillary dilatation |
| Ecocardiografia | Cardiac ultrasound (echocardiography) |
| Ecocardiografia doppler | Doppler echocardiography |
| Ecoencefalografia | Echoencephalography |
| Ecografia | Ultrasound (medical ultrasonography) |
| Ecografia addominale | Abdominal ultrasound |
| Ecografia colecisti e vie biliari | Ultrasound of the gallbladder and bile ducts |
| Ecografia della tiroide | Thyroid ultrasound |
| Ecografia epatica | Liver ultrasound |
| Ecografia mammaria | Breast ultrasound |
| Ecografia pancreatica | Pancreas ultrasound |
| Ecografia renale | Renal ultrasound |
| Elettrocardiografia | Electrocardiography (ECG) |
| Elettroencefalografia | Electroencephalography (EEG) |
| Elettroforesi delle sieroproteine | Serum protein electrophoresis |
| Elettromiografia | Electromyography (EMG) |
| Elettroneurografia | Electroneurography |
| Elettroretinografia | Electroretinography |
| Ematocrito | Hematocrit |
| Emocoltura | Blood culture |
| Emocromo (analisi del sangue, esame emocromocitometrico) | Complete blood count |
| Endoscopia | Endoscopy |
| Enteroscopia | Enteroscopy |
| Ergometria (ECG sotto sforzo) | Ergometry test |
| Esame chimico di succo gastrico | Gastric juice chemical examination |
| Esame del fundus oculi | Dilated fundus examination |
| Esame della mammella | Breast examination |
| Esame delle urine peso specifico | Urine specific gravity |
| Esame ginecologico | Gynecological examination |

| | |
|---|---|
| Esami di laboratorio | Laboratory tests |
| Esami sierologici | Serology blood tests |
| Esofagogastroduodenoscopia | Esophagogastroduodenoscopy |
| Esplorazione rettale | Rectal examination |
| Flebografia | Phlebography |
| Fluoroscopia | Fluoroscopy |
| Fosfatasi alcalina totale | Alkaline phosphatase |
| Gastroscopia | Gastroscopy |
| Glucosio nelle urine | Glucose urine test |
| Gonioscopia | Gonioscopy |
| HbsAg (antigene di superficie dell'epatite B) | HbsAg (Hepatitis B surface antigen) |
| Imaging a risonanza magnetica (risonanza magnetica tomografica) | Magnetic resonance imaging (MRI) |
| Indagini radiologiche del colon con clisma opaco a doppio contrasto | Barium enema |
| Isterosalpingografia | Hysterosalpingography |
| Isteroscopia | Hysterescopy |
| Laboratorio | Laboratory (lab) |
| Laparoscopia | Laparoscopy |
| Laringoscopia | Laryngoscopy |
| Linfangiografia (linfografia) | Lymphography (lymphangiography) |
| Magnetoencefalografia | Magnetoencephalography (MEG) |
| Mammografia (mastografia) | Mammography |
| Manometria esofagea | Esophageal manometry |
| Mantoux test | Mantoux test (PPD test) |
| Marker tumorale | Tumor marker |
| Mediastinoscopia | Mediastinoscopy |
| Medicina nucleare | Radioisotope scanning (nuclear medicine) |
| Mezzo di contrasto | Contrast medium |
| Mielografia | Myelography |
| Mielografia lombare | Lumbar myelography |
| Mielografia sotto-occipitale | Suboccipital myelography |
| Misurazione del polso | Pulse monitoring |
| Misurazione della pressione arteriosa | Blood pressure monitoring |
| Oftalmoscopìa | Ophtalmoscopy |
| Otoscopia | Otoscopy |
| Patch test | Patch test |
| Pelvigrafia | Pelvigraphy |
| Pelvimetria | Pelvimetry |
| Perimetria | Perimetry |
| Pielografia retrograda | Retrograde pyelography |
| Pletismografia | Plethysmography |
| Pneumoencefalografia | Pneumoencephalography |
| Polisonnografia | Polysomnography (sleep study) |
| Pressione venosa centrale | Central venous pressure (CVP) |
| Proteine nelle urine | Urine protein test |
| Prova della benzidina | Benzidine stool test |
| Prova di Weber | Weber test |
| Punteggio del coma di Glasgow | Glasgow coma scale |
| Puntura lombare (rachicentesi) | Lumbar puncture |
| Puntura suboccipitale | Suboccipital puncture |
| Radiografia | X-ray (radiography) |
| Radiografia del torace | Chest X-ray |
| Radiografia della colonna vertebrale | Spine X-ray (spine radiography) |
| Radiografia dentale | Dental X-ray |
| Radiografia gastroduodenale con pasto baritato | Barium meal (upper gastrointestinal series) |
| Radiografia ossea | Bone X-ray (bone radiography) |
| Rettoscopia | Rectoscopy |
| Riflesso patellare | Patellar reflex |
| Rifrattometria | Refractometry |
| Risonanza magnetica funzionale | Functional magnetic resonance imaging (functional MRI) |
| Rose Waaler test | Rose Waaler test |
| Scintigrafia epatobiliare con tecnezio -99m | Hepatobiliary scintigraphy with technetium -99m |
| Scintigrafia ossea | Bone scintigraphy |
| Scintigrafia polmonare | Lung scintigraphy |
| Scintigrafia renale | Renal scintigraphy |
| Scintigrafia splenica con tecnezio -99m | Spleen scintigraphy with technetium -99m |
| Scintigrafia tiroidea | Thyroid scintigraphy |
| Semenogelasi (antigene prostatico specifico) | Prostate specific antigen |
| Seroalbumina | Serum albumin |
| Sialografia (scialografia) | Sialography |
| Sigmoidoscopia | Sigmoidoscopy |
| Spermiogramma | Semen analysis |
| Spirometria (pneumometria) | Spirometry (vital capacity test) |
| Tempo di protrombina | Prothrombin time |

| | |
|---|---|
| Tempo di tromboplastina parziale | Partial thromboplastin time (PTT) |
| Test alfa-fetoproteina | Alpha-fetoprotein test (AFP test) |
| Test alla fenolsulfonftaleina | Phenolsulfonphthalein test (PSP test) |
| Test biochimici di sangue | Biochemical blood tests |
| Test cutaneo per le allergie "prick test" | Skin allergy testing (prick test) |
| Test del respiro (urea breath test) | Urea breath test |
| Test della bilirubina | Serum bilirubin |
| Test della bromosulfaleina di funzionalità epatica | Bromsulphalein liver function test |
| Test di agglutinazione | Agglutination tests |
| Test di captazione tiroidea dello iodio 131 | Iodine-131 thyroid test |
| Test di Coombs indiretto | Indirect Coombs test |
| Test di funzionalità epatica | Liver function tests |
| Test di gravidanza | Pregnancy test |
| Test di ormoni tiroidei nel sangue | Thyroid blood tests |
| Test di Papanicolaou (Pap test) | Papanicolau test (Pap test) |
| Test orale di tolleranca al glucosio (OGTT, curva da carico orale di glucosio) | Oral glucose tolerance test (OGTT) |
| Test rapido dello streptococco | Rapid strep test |
| Timpanocentesi | Tympanocentesis |
| Timpanometria | Tympanometry |
| Tomografia | Tomography |
| Tomografia ad emissione di positroni | Positron emission tomography |
| Tomografia computerizzata (TC) | Computed tomography (CT) |
| Tonometria | Tonometry |
| Toracoscopia | Thoracoscopy |
| Ultrasuono ad alta intensità focalizzato | High intensity focused ultrasound |
| Urea clearance (clearance dell'urea) | Urea clearance test |
| Ureteroscopia | Ureteroscopy |
| Uretrografia | Urethrography |
| Urinocoltura | Urine culture |
| Urobilinogeno nelle urine | Urobilinogen in urine |
| Urografia | Pyelography |
| Urografia intravenosa (pielografia intravenosa) | Intravenous pyelography |
| Velocità di eritro-sedimentazione | Erythrocyte sedimentation rate |
| Ventricolografia | Ventriculography |
| Volume urinario residuo | Post-void residual urine volume |

| GRAVIDANZA ED OSTETRICIA | PREGNANCY AND OBSTETRICS |
|---|---|
| Aborto abituale | Habitual abortion (recurrent miscarriage) |
| Aborto spontaneo | Spontaneous abortion (miscarriage) |
| Amniocentesi | Amniocentesis |
| Amnios | Amniotic sac |
| Amnioscopia | Amnioscopy |
| Anomalie di sviluppo fetale (anomalie fetali) | Fetal anomalies (fetal abnormalities) |
| Anomalie uterine | Uterine anomalies |
| Aspiratore a vuoto | Vacuum extractor (ventouse) |
| Asportazione chirurgica dell'utero (isterectomia) | Surgical removal of the uterus (hysterectomy) |
| Assenza di mestruazioni (amenorrea) | Absence of menstrual period (amenorrhea) |
| Banca del seme | Sperm bank |
| Blastocisti | Blastocyst |
| Canale del parto | Birth canal |
| Capezzolo | Nipple |
| Cardiotocografia | Cardiotocography |
| Ciclo mestruale | Menstrual cycle |
| Clinica ostetrica | Maternity hospital |
| Collo | Neck |
| Complesso TORCH | TORCH infections |
| Concezione | Conception |
| Contrazioni del travaglio | Labor contractions |
| Cordocentesi | Cordocentesis |
| Coriocarcinoma | Choriocarcinoma |
| Corion (corio) | Chorion |
| Culatta (deretano) | Breech |
| Depressione post-partum | Postnatal depression (postpartum depression) |
| Diabete gestazionale | Gestational diabetes |
| Dilatazione della cervice uterina | Cervical dilation |
| Distacco di placenta (abruptio placentae) | Placental abruption |
| Dotto galattoforo | Lactiferous duct |

| | |
|---|---|
| Durata della gravidanza | Duration of pregnancy |
| Durata di contrazioni | Duration of contraction |
| Eclampsia | Eclampsia |
| Ecografia | Ultrasound (medical ultrasonography) |
| Edema | Edema |
| Eiaculazione | Ejaculation |
| Embrione | Embryo |
| Emorragia | Bleeding (haemorrhage) |
| Episiotomia | Episiotomy |
| Eritroblastosi fetale (malattia emolitica del neonato) | Hemolytic disease of the newborn |
| Espulsione del feto | Expulsion of the baby |
| Espulsione della placenta | Expulsion of placenta |
| Estrogeno placentare | Placental estrogen |
| False contrazioni (contrazioni di Braxton Hicks) | Braxton Hicks contractons |
| Farmaci abortivi | Abortifacients |
| Farmaco con lo scopo di arrestare le contrazioni uterine (tocolisi) | Medication that suppresses premature labor (tocolytic) |
| Fase del parto | Stage of birth |
| Febbre puerperale | Puerperal fever |
| Fecondazione assistita (fecondazione artificiale) | Artificial insemination |
| Fertilizzazione in vitro | In vitro fertilisation |
| Feto | Fetus |
| Fetoscopia | Fetoscopy |
| Follicolo di Graaf | Graafian follicle |
| Forcipe | Forceps |
| Frequenza di contrazioni uterine | Labor contraction frequency |
| Funicolo ombelicale | Umbilical cord |
| Gemelli | Twins |
| Gemelli fraterni (gemelli dizigoti) | Dizygotic twins (biovular twins) |
| Gemell i identici (gemelli monozigoti) | Monozygotic twins (identical twins) |
| Genitore | Parent |
| Genitore biologico | Biological parent |
| Ginecologia | Gynecology |
| Gonadotropina corionica | Chorion-gonadotrophin |
| Gravidanza (gestazione) | Pregnancy |
| Gravidanza ectopica | Ectopic pregnancy (extrauterine pregnancy) |
| Gravidanza gemellare | Multiple pregnancy |
| Imene | Hymen |
| Impianto | Implantation |
| Incubatrice | Incubator |
| Infezione | Infection |
| Infiammazione del sacco amniotico (corioamniosite) | Inflammation of the fetal membranes (chorioamnionitis) |
| Infiammazione della vescica urinaria (cistite) | Inflammation of the urinary bladder (cystitis) |
| Iniezione intracitoplasmatica dello spermatozoo | Intracytoplasmatic sperm injection |
| Intensità di contrazione | Intensity of contractions |
| Interruzione di gravidanza (aborto) | Abortion (pregnancy termination) |
| Iperemia dell'ovaio | Ovarian hyperemia |
| Iperplasia endometriale | Endometrial hyperplasia |
| Ipertensione arteriosa sistemica | High blood pressure (hypertension) |
| Ipertrofia dell'utero | Hypertrophy of uterus |
| Ipotrofia fetale | Fetal hypotrophy |
| Lattazione | Lactation |
| Liquido amniotico | Amniotic fluid |
| Lithopedion | Lithopedion (stone baby) |
| Lochi | Lochia |
| Lunghezza di neonato | Body length of a newborn |
| Macrosomia fetale | Macrosomia (big baby syndrome) |
| Madre | Mother |
| Malattia di Hirschsprung (ostruzione del colon congenita) | Meconium ileus |
| Mammella | Breast |
| Mastite puerperale | Puerperal mastitis |
| Meconio | Meconium |
| Menopausa | Menopause |
| Mestruazione | Menstruation |
| Microcefalia | Microcephaly |
| Mifepristone | Mifepristone |
| Morula | Morula |
| Mucosa interna dell'utero (endometrio) | Inner membrane of the uterus (endometrium) |
| Nato morto | Stillborn |
| Nausea | Nausea |
| Neonato | Newborn (infant) |
| Neonato pretermine | Preterm newborn |
| Neonatologia | Neonatology |
| Ombelico | Navel (belly button) |
| Ostetrica (levatrice) | Midwife |
| Ostetricia | Obstetrics |
| Ostetrico | Obstetrician |

| | |
|---|---|
| Ovaia (ovario) | Ovary |
| Ovidotto (ovidutto) | Fallopian tube (oviduct) |
| Ovodonazione | Egg donation |
| Ovogenesi | Oogenesis |
| Ovulazione | Ovulation |
| Padre | Father |
| Pannolino | Diaper |
| Parto | Childbirth |
| Parto a termine | Full term birth |
| Parto nell'acqua | Water birth |
| Parto patologico | Pathological birth |
| Parto post-termine | Postmature birth |
| Parto pretermine | Premature birth |
| Parto prolungato | Prolonged birth |
| Pelvi ristretto | Contracted pelvis |
| Pelvimetria | Pelvimetry |
| Peritonite da meconio | Meconium peritonitis |
| Peso di neonato | Fetal weight (birth mass) |
| pH-metria fetale | Fetal pH-metry |
| Pielonefrite | Pyelonephritis |
| Placenta | Placenta |
| Placenta accreta | Placenta accreta |
| Placenta previa | Placenta previa |
| Plagiocefalia | Plagiocephaly |
| Pluripara | Multigravida |
| Pompa tiralatte | Breast pump |
| Posizione del feto trasversale | Transverse fetal position |
| Posizione podalica del feto | Breech position |
| Preeclampsia (gestosi) | EPH gestosis (pre-eclampsia) |
| Primipara | Primigravida |
| Procreazione assistita | Medically assisted procreation |
| Produzione di saliva eccessiva (ipersalivazione) | Excessive secretion of saliva (hypersalivation) |
| Profilo biofisico fetale | Biophysical profile of the fetus |
| Progesterone | Progesterone |
| Progesterone placentare | Placental progesterone |
| Prolasso del funicolo ombelicale | Umbilical cord prolapse |
| Prolattina | Prolactin |
| Psicosi post-partum | Postpartum psychosis |
| Puerperio | Postnatal (postpartum period, puerperium) |
| Quattro gemelli | Quadruplets |
| Raschiamento (curetage) | Curettage |
| Respirazione | Breathing |
| Rischio teratogenico | Pregnancy risk factors |
| Ritenzione urinaria | Urinary retention (ischuria) |
| Rottura delle membrane | Rupture of membranes |
| Rottura precoce delle membrane | Premature rupture of membranes |
| Sala parto | Delivery room |
| Segno del Chadwick (tinta bluastra alla vagina) | Chadwick's sign |
| Seme (sperma) | Semen (sperm) |
| Sepsi puerperale | Puerperal sepsis |
| Sindrome da aspirazione di meconio | Meconium aspiration syndrome |
| Sindrome del terzo giorno (baby blues) | Maternity blues (baby blues) |
| Sopravvivenza di spermatozoo | Sperm viability |
| Spermatozoo | Spermatozoon (sperm cell) |
| Spingere | Push |
| Sterilità | Infertility |
| Surrogazione di maternità | Surrogate mother (womb mother) |
| Suzione | Suckling |
| Tagliare (intersecare) | Cut |
| Taglio cesareo | Cesarean section (C-section) |
| Testa | Head |
| Translucenza nucale | Nuchal scan (nuchal translucency) |
| Uovo | Ovum |
| Utero | Womb (uterus) |
| Vagina | Vagina |
| Varici degli arti inferiori | Leg varicose veins |
| Villi coriali | Chorionic villi |
| Villocentesi | Chorionic villus sampling |
| Vomito (emetismo) | Vomiting |

ABOUT THE AUTHOR

Edita Ciglenečki is medical translator with Academic degrees in Biomedical Sciences and Public Health Sciences. Besides Croatian, being her mother tongue, she is a holder of international diplomas in English, French and Italian language. For many years she worked as a medical professional inside the travel industry. This dictionary is the product of her own working experience built on her passion for travelling, medicine and language skills.

www.ingramcontent.com/pod-product-compliance
Lightning Source LLC
Chambersburg PA
CBHW070105210526
45170CB00013B/745